Therapeutic Communications for Health Professionals

2nd Edition

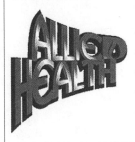

Therapeutic Communications for Health Professionals

2nd Edition

Carol D. Tamparo, BS, PhD, CMA-A
Dean, Business and Allied Health
Lake Washington Technical College
Kirkland, Washington

Wilburta Q. Lindh, CMA
Medical Assistant Program Coordinator
Highline Community College
DesMoines, Washington

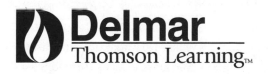

Delmar
Thomson Learning™

Notice to the Reader

Cover Design: Brucie Rosch

Delmar Staff

Publisher: William Brottmiller
Acquisitions Editor: Marlene Pratt
Developmental Editor: Helen Yackel
Production Coordinator: James Zayicek
Art and Design Coordinator: Richard Killar
Project Editor: William Trudell

Library of Congress Cataloging-in-Publication Data
Tamparo, Carol D., 1940–
      Therapeutic communications for health professionals / Carol D.
   Tamparo, Wilburta Q. Lindh. — 2nd ed.
          p.   cm.
      Prev. ed. has title: Therapeutic communications for allied health
   professions.
      Includes bibliographical references and index.
      ISBN 0-7668-0921-8
      1. Allied health personnel and patient Examinations, questions,
   etc. 2. Interpersonal communication Examinations, questions, etc.
   I. Tamparo, Carol D.   Therapeutic communications for allied health
   professions.   II. Lindh, Wilburta Q.   III. Title.
   R727.3.T36 2000
   610.69'6—dc21   99-33170
                                                        CIP

Printed in Canada

Table of Contents

Preface   ix

Section I   *Therepeutic Communications*   1

Chapter 1   **Self-Awareness**   3
Human and Technical Relations Skills   6
Social and Therapeutic Communications   7
The Therapeutic Process   9
What is Your Style?   15
Professional Application   16

Chapter 2   **Basic Communication Skills**   23
Communication Cycle   25
Verbal Communications   28
Nonverbal Communications   29
Word of Caution   33
Communication with Diverse Populations   34
Influence of Technology on Communication   35
Team Communication   36
Listening Skills   36

Chapter 3   **The Helping Interview**   45
Interview Components   46
Orientation   48
Identification of Problem   50
Levels of Need   52
Questioning Techniques   52
Roadblocks to Communication   54
Resolution of the Problem   58

Chapter 4   **Defense Mechanisms**   69
Regression   70
Repression   71
Sublimation   72
Projection   72
Displacement   72
Undoing   73
Compensation   73
Identification   73
Denial   73
Rationalization   74

Section II   *Learning Theories of Growth and Development*   **77**

Chapter 5   **Cognitive Development Learning Theory**   **79**
Jean Piaget (1896–1980)   80

Chapter 6   **Psychoanalytic Development Learning Theories**   **89**
Sigmund Freud (1856–1939)   90
Eric Erikson (1902–1994)   95

Chapter 7   **Moral Development Learning Theories**   **107**
Piaget's Six Dimensions of Moral Development   108
Lawrence Kohlberg's Stages
   of Moral Development   109
Role of Health Professionals   110

Chapter 8   **Behavioral and Humanistic Learning Theories**   **115**
Ivan Pavlov, Behaviorist   116
B.F. Skinner, Behaviorist   118
Social Learning Theory   119
Abraham Maslow, Humanist   119
Conclusion   121

Section III   *The Therapeutic Response*   **125**

Chapter 9   **The Therapeutic Response in Age Groups**   **127**
Children   128
Adolescents   130
Adults   133
Elder Adults   135

Chapter 10   **The Therapeutic Response to Frightened,**
   Angry, and Aggressive Clients   **147**
The Frightened Client   148
The Angry/Aggressive Client   150
The Therapeutic Response   152

Chapter 11   **The Therapeutic Response to Stressed**
   and Anxious Clients   **157**
What is Stress?   158
Stress Theories   159
Anxiety   162
Stress and the Life Cycle   164
How to Reduce Stress   169

Chapter 12	**The Therapeutic Response to Depressed Clients**	**175**
	Types of Depression	177
	Depression and the Life Cycle	182
	Therapeutic Approaches	183
Chapter 13	**The Therapeutic Response to Suicidal Clients**	**187**
	Suicide: Statistics & Risk Factors	188
	Four Stages of Contemplating Suicide	190
	The Therapeutic Response	191
Chapter 14	**The Therapeutic Response to Sexually Suggestive Clients**	**197**
	Attitudes Toward Sexuality	198
	Therapeutic Approaches	199
Chapter 15	**The Therapeutic Response to Drug-Dependent Clients**	**203**
	Introduction	204
	Alcoholism	205
	Abuse of Other Drugs	207
	The Therapeutic Response	210
Chapter 16	**The Therapeutic Response to Abusive and Abused Clients**	**213**
	Introduction	214
	Phases of Violence	215
	Types of Abuse	216
	Rape	219
	Physical Indicators of Abuse	220
	The Therapeutic Response	222
Chapter 17	**The Therapeutic Response to AIDS Clients**	**227**
	Introduction	228
	The Realities of AIDS	231
	The Therapeutic Response	233
Chapter 18	**The Therapeutic Response to Clients Experiencing Loss, Grief, Dying, and Death**	**237**
	Introduction	239
	G.L. Engle	239
	Kübler-Ross	239
	Cultural Influences on Grief and Death	240
	Kinds of Losses	240
	Factors That Influence Grief	241
	The Right to Die	245
Glossary		**251**
Index		**255**

Preface

When there is dissatisfaction, distrust, or displeasure in the professional relationship between health care professionals and the clients they serve, it is usually the result of very poor or nontherapeutic communications rather than the lack of technical skills. If you are reading this material it is because you or someone else realized the absolute necessity for superior therapeutic communication skills. Without these skills, clients — who have the ultimate power in the relationship — will simply seek care elsewhere.

We wrote this material because of our sense that therapeutic communication skills are necessary for any health care professional. The practical illustrations along with the basic fundamentals of growth and development and communication skills make this text as versatile as it is useful.

Organization

This material has three major sections: Therapeutic Communications, Learning Theories of Growth and Development, and The Therapeutic Response. The section on Therapeutic Communictions will introduce you to basic communication skills and the helping interview. You will be more aware of your own communication style and how to respond to others. The section on Learning Theories of Growth and Development provides background information on several theories that help you to better understand yourself and those you serve. The third section suggests appropriate therapeutic communications for specific populations. A table of contents will facilitate ease in using one module independent of the other two. A comprehensive glossary of terms appears at the end of the text.

Measurable objectives that clearly identify the chapter's goals and objectives are presented at the beginning of every chapter. At the end of each chapter there are exercises, many of which are reflective and introspective in nature. Some exercises are designed for class participation; others are for personal use. Becoming skilled in therapeutic communications is a lifelong process. There is always more to learn about human behavior and relationships. This material provides a basis for reference as you begin the process of therapeutic communications.

Features

The fingerprints scattered throughout the material are used to provide a mental picture, a memory boost, and a touch of humor to the material. Duuana Otey has been the original illustrator for the fingerprints. Our many thanks to the Delmar's illustrator who took Duuana's original illustrations along with our ideas to create the final product. We hope they will help you remember the material and bring a smile to your face.

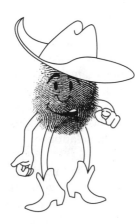

"I'll help you be therapeutic."

New to This Edition

Consideration of the great impact of the electronic age and its influence on communication has been given. Additional references to diversity issues and transcultural experiences are included in Chapter 2. Team communication, so important to today's health care, is highlighted. Seasonal affective disorder and postpartum depression are discussed in Chapter 12. Many chapter exercises will suggest the use of computer technology through access to the Internet.

Support Materials

The Instructor's Manual will include classroom exercises, sample examination questions, and practical suggestions that have been helpful to the authors in their classroom experience.

About the Authors

Carol D. Tamparo, B.S., Ph.D., CMA-A, is a graduate of the University of Wyoming and the Union Institute. She is the Dean of Business and Allied Health at Lake Washington Technical College in Kirkland, Washington. She is the coauthor of *Medical Law, Ethics, and Bioethics for Ambulatory Care, 4th Edition, Diseases of the Human Body, 4th Edition,* and *Delmar's Comprehensive Medical Assisting, Administrative and Clinical Competencies.*

Wilburta (Billie) Lindh, A.A., CMA, is a graduate of the Medical Assistant Program of Highline Community College, Des Moines, Washington. Currently, she is the director of this department, which involves teaching responsibilities and coordination of courses for Medical Reception and Medical Transcription programs. Billie is the coauthor of *The Radiology Word Book, The Ophthalmology Word Book,* and *Delmar's Comprehensive Medical Assisting, Administrative and Clinical Competencies.*

Acknowledgements

Each of us has not only sensed importance of therapeutic communications in health care, we have attempted to always practice the techniques in our personal and professional lives. Students provided examples for us, and tested the material in the classroom. The personal experiences that came from immediate and extended family members, colleagues, and friends provide the basis for the stories and scenarios included in this text. We are grateful for their sharing of these often personal and painful examples.

The professional assistance given by the Delmar staff was helpful, supportive, and much appreciated.

We give special thanks to the reviewers who helped contribute extensively to the development of this second edition.

Brenda Foster, MS, CMA, ART
East Tennessee State University
Elizabethton, Tennessee

Annette Torres, RMA, CPT
National School of Technology
North Miami Beach, Florida

Debra Schmidt-Shafer, BSN, RN
Blair College
Colorado Springs, Colorado

Marge Hinkemyer, RN, BS, MA
St. Cloud Technical College
St. Cloud, Minnesota

Jean Griffith, BS
North Central O.I.C
Barrackville, West Virginia

Julie Hosley, RN, CMA
Carteret Community College
Morehead City, North Carolina

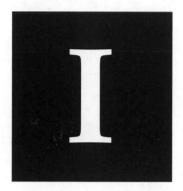

Therapeutic Communications

Chapter 1

Self-Awareness

Procedural Goal

To assist the student in realizing the importance of self-awareness and to understand its effect on interpersonal communication.

Learning Objectives

Upon completion of this unit, when given a written examination, the student will respond to the following with a minimum of ____% (percent to be determined by instructor) accuracy within the defined class period for the exam.

- List at least two characteristics of human relations skills.
- Compare/contrast social and therapeutic communications.
- Define self-awareness.
- Describe at least five influences on perception.
- Identify two reasons to enter into self-analysis.
- Differentiate between the "ideal self," the "public self," and the "real self."
- Describe the Johari Window and its use in self-analysis.

- Identify techniques for modifying negative characteristics.
- List at least six questions to ask yourself before you enter into a helping profession.

An elderly woman, Mrs. Nelson, was attacked by a German shepherd while walking her toy poodle. The German shepherd came out from the yard, where it was usually restrained, attacking Mrs. Nelson and her poodle on the sidewalk. Serious injuries resulted.

Before the owner could call the shepherd, Mrs. Nelson had been pushed onto the pavement falling backward striking her head. A deep, five-inch laceration was made in the back of the skull, and heavy bleeding resulted. There were two puncture wounds in her ring finger from the dog's bite. The finger was fractured in two places. In the emergency room, she would discover that she also had a fractured coccyx. The toy poodle, also seriously injured, survived surgery at the emergency veterinary clinic.

Mrs. Nelson was treated with care and compassion in an overcrowded emergency room on a Sunday night. More than one nurse, the emergency room physician, and the staff members in the hospital lab and the x-ray department were all involved in her care. Several efforts failed to stop the bleeding. It was several hours before Mrs. Nelson was released to go home with her finger in splint, her head wound sutured, and a very tight bandage around her head.

She was not able to sleep from her pain and discomfort, and worry about her poodle at the emergency veterinary clinic. She was advised to see her personal physician the next morning for a blood test and to return in three days either to the emergency room or to her physician to have the stitches removed.

Her family called and took her to her personal physician the next morning, with her emergency room records in hand. The medical office assistant told Mrs. Nelson she would have to wait because the doctor did not see patients without prior appointments in the morning. Mrs. Nelson explained that the emergency room physician said it was important the test be run in the morning. After more than an hour, her physician agreed to see her and perform the blood test.

The personal physician seemed irritated by this interruption in the day's schedule, checked the head wound and the finger, and asked the assistant to redress the wound. The woman's hair was badly matted with dried and caked blood, and the assistant seemed uneasy about touching the woman's head or hair. However, she placed a new bandage on the woman's head and released her with no instructions to return. The bandage was so loose that it fell off in the afternoon.

Mrs. Nelson hoped that her personal physician would appreciate the concern the emergency room physician had for her red blood cell count. She hoped to be able to discuss her fears and anxieties, have her questions answered, and be given some assurance about recovery. At that time, Mrs. Nelson's emotional needs were greater than her need for technical medical care. When it was time to return to have the stitches removed, where do you suppose Mrs. Nelson went?

She returned to the hospital where she had been treated with care and concern. She was becoming embarrassed about the dried blood in her hair and the instructions not to get the wound wet, so the assistant who helped the physician remove the stitches gently used a warm wash cloth and peroxide to remove most of the dried blood. The physician told her the head and finger wounds were healing nicely, but that the coccyx fracture would cause her discomfort for quite some time. Mrs. Nelson left the hospital a little less traumatized, knowing it would be several weeks before she would feel like herself again. But she felt like she and her unfortunate accident were unimportant to her personal physician.

Three months after the accident, Mrs. Nelson needed a physician's summary of her recovery process and any expected complications for insurance purposes. She returned to her primary care physician who said, "There is nothing I can do for you now. Your head wound has healed nicely. You saw the orthopedic surgeon about your finger. I have no idea how long you will have pain from the coccyx fracture, and neither does any other physician."

Still uncomfortable about her primary care physician's response, she chose to see another physician. In her interview with the new physician, the verbal exchange turned to the accident. The physician leaned forward seeking out Mrs. Nelson's concern and said, "Gosh, tell me what happened." In less than ten minutes, she poured out her story.

Recognizing the need to be therapeutic, the physician asked, "How is your dog?" He also commented, "It certainly seems to me that you should be able to safely walk your dog on a public sidewalk." He then proceeded to examine her.

Technically, this physician could do no more for the woman than either her primary care physician or the emergency room physician. What this physician did do is listen to her, acknowledge her trauma, verify that she was not at fault, and assure her that any medical needs would be cared for to the best of his ability.

———————

This scenario describes an actual ordeal. It illustrates both positive and negative therapeutic communication and human relations skills. In this module, you will become more aware of how your personal perceptions affect your communication style. You will be asked to complete exercises to assist you in becoming proficient in the skills necessary for therapeutic communication.

Human and Technical Relations Skills

When you interact with people, you engage in human relations. Human relations skills, sometimes referred to as interpersonal skills, are employed in both personal and professional relationships. Some situations will be pleasant and fun; others will be unpleasant, strained, and unsatisfactory. Human relations skills include verbal and nonverbal communications, such as how you communicate and whether you are aware of the effect you have on others, how you dress and take care of yourself, the language you use, and even how you feel about yourself.

An example of human relations skills form the scenario is the care and compassionate treatment Mrs. Nelson received at the emergency room as contrasted to the irritation about the disruption of the schedule and impersonal treatment she received from the physician office personnel.

Technical skills represent those specialized skills that are required to support and deliver professional medical care. The preceding scenario illustrates several technical skills demonstrated by the staff in the emergency room, that is, the lab and x-ray staff support, and the assistant who bandaged the wounds and then performed the follow-up visit care by using the warm wash cloth and peroxide to remove most of the dried blood from Mrs. Nelson's hair.

In the ambulatory care setting, neither human relations skills nor technical skills are sufficient by themselves. You must have a combination of the two.

Social and Therapeutic Communications

Human relations skills are translated into social and therapeutic communications when there is contact with persons seeking attention. Social communication requires nonspecific professional skills. For instance, you may offer assistance to an elderly gentleman removing his coat in the office, or you may dry the tears of a child who has just had an injection.

Therapeutic communication requires specific, well-defined professional skills. When you instruct a client regarding preparation for a flexible sigmoidoscopy, or when you explain the billing procedures to a new client, specific, well-defined professional skills are used.

Therapeutic communication takes place between a person who has a specific need and a person who is skilled in techniques that can alleviate or diminish that problem. As in human relations skills, however, how you feel about yourself will directly affect how successful you are in social and therapeutic communications.

A number of influences greatly impact our lives and dominate how we feel about ourselves and how we feel others perceive us. A few of these influences are listed for you.

Genetic Influences

We all inherit physical traits from our ancestors. Our height, body structure, and skin color are defined and established by the genes passed on during fertilization. There is very little we can do to change our basic body's bone structure or skin color. Even the fact that we are male or female influences how we feel about ourselves and how others perceive us.

Cultural Influences

Every culture has its own customs and traditions. These will have a direct influence on the person we are and how we are perceived. The traditional greeting in Japan is to bow at the waist. In other countries, the greeting is to extend the right hand for a handshake. Some cultures dictate that clothing is worn to cover the body; other cultures believe clothing is a burden and unnecessary. Much emphasis is placed on attire in this country. How would you be accepted if you choose to walk in town wearing only a loin cloth? And how strange would you feel in parts of Africa in a three-piece suit?

Economic Influences

The financial status of our family relates directly to the type of education and life experiences we share. These influence our being and mold us to the person we are. If you were born and raised in poverty, your perception of life and others is likely to be much different than if you were born and raised in affluence. Exposure to the fine arts and the opportunity to travel extensively impacts our diversity.

Internal Milieu

Each of us has a very individualized and specialized body. Some of us may be taking drugs/medications that either replace or enhance the hormones produced by the body and its functions. Many individuals, because of injury or disease, must live with chronic pain. The visibly disabled are perceived differently than those with a hidden disability or no disability. The ways in which we handle these diversities to a great extent is governed by our internal milieu.

Educational Experience

As the mind expands and new approaches and theories are investigated, our lives are changed and molded into different patterns. Those who have not finished high school may have a different perception from those who finish college. Those who have trained in the military or in an apprenticeship or have received on-the-job training will have a variety of opportunities different from others.

Life Experience

Life experiences teach us much. Those who have experienced grief and loss react differently from those who have not. Experiencing a separation or divorce has a great impact on the way you view future relationships and on your level of trust in others. Whether life's trials have been fairly easy or very harsh for you will influence your lifestyle.

Spiritual Influences

Your spiritual beliefs influence how you feel about yourself and how you are perceived by others. Do you have a belief in a supreme being? Have you been or are you currently involved in organized religion? Do you feel you need religion or is it just a crutch, a myth, or something you have no interest in whatsoever. Or do you have a faith that is encouraging and uplifting and gives you hope?

Values/Morals

Values or morals are rules we live by or habits of conduct. Values are attributes that are important to us in relation to self and others. What are your values? What is your work ethic? Have there been influences in your life that encouraged pride and self-actualization or did the influences promote a "why me? poor me!" attitude?

Models/Mentors

Models are found in national leaders, "Superman," "Rambo," parents, teachers, spiritual leaders, and public figures. They are persons for whom we have a deep respect. They are doing or being something we wish we could do or be. Models are both positive and negative and have a powerful influence over a long period of time.

"The Electronic Age"

Today, most of us are spending a greater part of the day being influenced directly by electronic media. Electronic media may include television, video and film interactions, telecommunications, computers, the Internet with its chat rooms, bulletin boards, and e-mail. The influence of **cyberspace** has not yet reached its full potential nor has its effects on human relations been fully understood. Most of the world is getting "turned on" or "plugged in" to the Electronic Age and will be directly influenced by its effects.

The Therapeutic Process

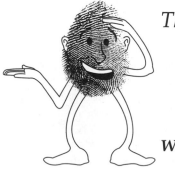

"I'm in search of myself. Have you seen me recently?"

To begin the therapeutic process we must learn to recognize and evaluate our own actions and responses in given situations. It is important to know how we feel about ourselves. We must understand ourselves and like ourselves before we can begin to understand and like others.

What is Self-Awareness?

Self-awareness is being aware of oneself as an individual (Figure 1-1). It is all the beliefs a person has with respect to behavior. It is our mental image of ourselves. It may be realistic or

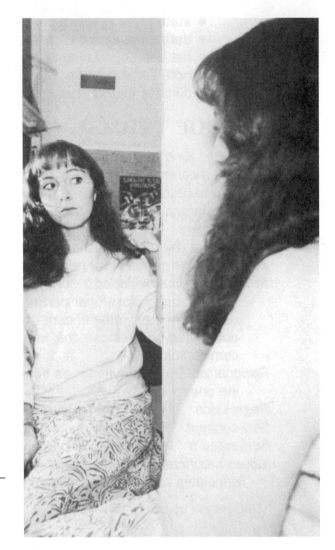

Figure 1-1

"When you look in the mirror, do you see a person who finds much satisfaction in life, or someone who focuses on negative experiences?"

unrealistic. It is changeable and is affected by life experiences. Their self-awareness begins to form at a very early age and is well established by the age of six.

Before going further, take time now to complete the **self-analysis** questions in Exercise 1 and the "I am" statements in Exercise 2 in this chapter. These exercises are designed to stimulate thinking about yourself and to assist you in making some assessments about your level of **self-acceptance**. What did you learn about yourself? Do you accept yourself as you are now or would you like to make some changes?

TO BE FULLY ME
I need to remember
I am me
and in all the world
there is no one
like me.

I give myself permission
to discover me and use me
lovingly

I look at myself and see
a beautiful instrument
in which that can happen.
I love me
I appreciate me
I value me.

Virginia Satir[1]

While we can not do much to change these influences, we can recognize their presence, evaluate their effect, and begin to initiate change where possible. One way to do this is through self-analysis.

The Value of Self-Analysis

The value in self-analysis is the fact that it helps us determine who we are as seen by self and by others. It is a tool to show us how to be aware of both positive and negative characteristics so that changes may be implemented. These changes bring about growth and keep us from becoming stagnant. Whether we like it or not, we are always changing. Self-awareness helps give us the power to accept or possibly alter these changes.

Each of us has three selves living within one body: The ideal self, the public self, and the real self. The *ideal self* is the person we think we should be. Our parents, peers, and influential people in our lives tell us to "conform" to what is socially acceptable. The ideal self represents the person we would like to be someday. The *Public Self* is how we want others to see us. There may be many public selves depending upon the circle of people with whom we have contact. For example, our public self is the image we want others to have about us. In other words, it is our reputation. The *Real Self* is the inner, natural self. It is authentic and spontaneous. When you are most true to yourself and transparent to others, you are being your real self.

In order to have positive self-acceptance, there must be congruency between all three selves. All three must be balanced and we must feel good about each dimension of ourselves.

Complete the exercise related to the three selves to assist you in determining how you personally feel about the three dimensions of yourself. Now that you have completed the exercise, do some self-analysis. What did you learn about yourself from this project? Are you willing to make any changes in your life to accommodate growth? What kinds of opportunities can you think of that would help you achieve these changes?

Johari Window

As you continue to ponder on your ideal self, public self, and real self, the theory of the **Johari Window** in Figures 1-2 and 1-3 may reveal some useful information about yourself. Joseph Luft and Harry Ingham chose a four-paned window to illustrate the human personality. Each pane of the window represents a segment of self. The panes are presented on the following pages.[2]

The goal of the Johari Window is to make the "open" section of your window the largest section so that communication flows freely among confident people who are unafraid of making a mistake and facing rejection. Your goal is to seek feedback from others, especially in the "blind" pane so that you are more aware of yourself and open to others. Listen carefully to what others say about your "blind" areas. Be willing to accept their perceptions and suggestions. Examine what is "hidden" in your window. Risk revealing to a close friend some of that information. You will find life more joyous and satisfying. The goal is to strive for a window that has the "open" area as its largest area.

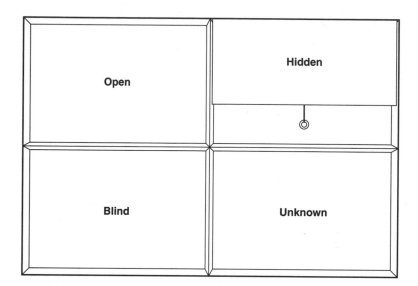

Figure 1-2 Johari Window with Small Open Frame

Open:	This window pane is characterized by a free and open exchange of known information between yourself and others.
Hidden:	The information in this pane is known by you, but for one reason or another, you keep this information hidden from others. You may fear that if others knew this information, they would feel differently about you.
	As your relationship with another develops, you may choose to reveal hidden information as your trust level deepens.
Blind:	This pane contains information is obvious to others, but not to you; it might include mannerisms, the way you say things, or the style you use to relate to others.
	Feedback from others will increase your knowledge regarding this window pane.
Unknown:	This section is unknown both to self and to others. Some of this information may be so far below the surface that no one will ever be aware of it.
	The more we use self-analysis, and the more honest we can be with ourselves, the smaller this window pane will become.

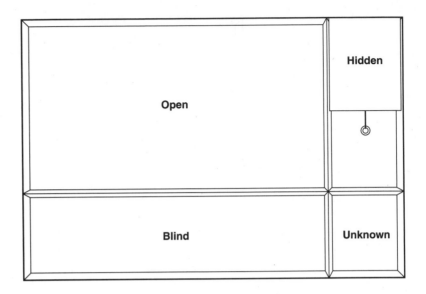

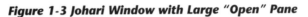

Figure 1-3 Johari Window with Large "Open" Pane

NEW POSSIBILITIES

Give your body a message of love and value.
We have many, many parts to ourselves that are
present, but not manifest...
present, but unknown to us...
present, but covered up.

So our journey onward,
regardless of where we are,
can always be
a delicious surprise.
Sometimes with pain,
Sometimes with excitement,
But always with new possibilities
for ourselves.

Virginia Satir[3]

What is Your Style?

Who are you?

On the sheet provided for you in Exercise 4 at the end of this section, identify five positive characteristics and five negative characteristics about yourself. Stop now in your reading and perform this exercise.

Did you have difficulty identifying five positive characteristics about yourself while you felt the list of negative characteristics could go on and on? What does that tell you about yourself? Do you have a positive attitude and think you have some really great qualities? Or are you feeling you have little worth and are a failure? If you have negative characteristics that you feel could be changed, there are ways to make that possible. Learn to identify your strengths and use them to their fullest. Also, identify your weak traits and habits and begin to nibble away at changing them into positive traits.

It is important, however, to recognize that each of us is a unique and wonderful individual who is special and important. It is essential to acknowledge that we are all different and that difference does not make us right or wrong, good or bad.

What to Do About Negative Discoveries

After careful analysis of the exercises provided in this section, you will have undoubtedly discovered many positive characteristics about yourself. And yes, you probably also discovered some negative characteristics as well. Do not be discouraged by the negative. Rather use these traits as stepping stones on which to build new positive traits. Examine the negative traits and write replacement positive traits next to them. Consciously be aware of your responses during interactions with others and practice using the new positive traits.

There are many self-help materials available today. Take a trip to the library and check out one or two books and begin a reading project to learn how to turn negative characteristics into positives. You may choose to investigate counseling or therapy groups to assist with this process. Look for those positive models and/or mentors who can provide assistance.

Many find it helpful to analyze why they respond the way they do during situations. For example, the person who is very bossy may be experiencing insecurity. To remedy this negative trait, consciously allow others to make suggestions. Remember that it is not essential to be in control all the time. It is all right to allow others to have some authority in decision-making processes. By sharing the responsibility and the direction to be taken, others feel they have opportunity for input and the working relationship will be much more efficient.

Professional Application

After reflecting on yourself and how you relate to others and considering ways to become better at human relations and therapeutic communications, there is an important concept for consideration. Are you the best kind of person to be in a helping profession? Is your personality suitable for such a career choice? Will your own needs, desires, and capabilities be suitable or detrimental to the needs of others?

Some members of helping professions, women particularly, give so much of themselves to their clients and their work that they quickly become disillusioned and suffer burnout. Others remain so aloof and detached from their work and clients' needs that they can become rude and disinterested. Neither description is appropriate nor successful.

There are some questions for you to keep in mind. Ask yourself the following simple questions:

1. *Do you genuinely enjoy helping people in a therapeutic manner?* This implies that you have the technical skills and knowledge to help people solve their problems, and that you do so without the need to create more power for yourself.

2. *Can you feel comfortable assuming a "servant" role for those in need?* Servant does not imply slave, but you must genuinely enjoy serving the needs of others.

3. *Will you always be able to treat any person as a "guest" no matter what their special circumstances may be?* You must keep in mind that your employment is dependent upon a satisfied customer.

4. *Can you be open to people and accept their differences?* Even though your personal lifestyle might be quite the opposite, can you be accepting and unflappable? Are you tolerant? Can you keep your opinions to yourself?

5. *Can you be firm, yet gentle?* Procedures you perform may cause discomfort and/or pain, but your verbal and nonverbal communication must convey both firmness and gentleness.

6. *Can you keep yourself out of a codependent relationship with those you help?* People in helping professions may adopt a hostile attitude toward their clients after so many years of rescuing and giving so much. Many health care professionals are harried and overcommitted and so locked into a caretaker role that they feel dismayed and rejected when they cannot "save" someone. Many books are available that can be most helpful in recognizing codependency. It is the authors' belief that an understanding of codependency and how it can interfere with therapeutic communication is important for anyone in a helping, therapeutic profession.

Exercise 1

Complete the following questions to help assess a positive self-acceptance or a negative self-acceptance.

1. Am I secure enough not to let others make me feel guilty? Often? Some of the time? Rarely? Never?

2. Do I worry needlessly?

3. Do I understand my failures and still feel okay?

4. Do I feel equal, not inferior or superior, to others?

5. Do I feel valuable? Often? Some of the time? Rarely? Never?

6. Do I feel needed? Often? Some of the time? Rarely? Never?

7. Do I feel I deserve compliments? How do I respond when someone compliments me?

8. Do I accept praise and give compliments graciously?

9. Do I resist others who try to dominate me?

10. Do I make judgments and/or decisions on my own?

11. Do I allow myself to acknowledge my feelings?

Exercise 2

Read the following statements and select the ten statements you think best describe you. Then select eight statements you think least describe you.

"I AM" STATEMENTS

I am a perfectionist.

I am reserved.

I am a happy person.

I am easily hurt.

I am self-conscious.

I am sympathetic.

I am unpredictable.

I am creative.

I am naive.

I am self-sacrificing.

I am able to live by rules.

I am shy.

I have a good self-image.

I am hard to get along with.

I am ambitious.

I am an understanding person.

I am easygoing.

I am often lonely.

I am socially inept.

I am a well-groomed person.

I am selfish.

I am not very attractive.

I am precise.

I am overprotective.

I am tolerant.

I am a people person.

I am fickle.

I am fun-loving.

I am demanding of myself.

I am generally trusting.

I am oversensitive.

I am dependable.

I am realistic.

I am well liked.

I am impulsive.

I am secure.

I am able to express emotions.

I am often opinionated.

I am self-reliant.

I am sometimes incompetent.

I am generous.

I am a worrier.

I am intelligent.

I am afraid of failure.

I am competitive.

I am courageous.

I am often depressed.

I am socially adept.

I am in control.

I am disorganized.

I am an attractive person.

I am a decision maker.

I am usually confident.

I am realistic.

I am energetic.

I am responsible for myself.

I am assertive.

I am argumentative.

I am often suspicious of others.

I often feel insecure.

I can usually make a decision.

I am poised.

Exercise 3

Using the columns provided, list adjectives that describe how you perceive your three selves.

Ideal Self	Public Self	Real Self
Ask the question, what kind of person do I wish to become?	You may wish to ask someone who knows you to describe you.	What do you really feel inside?

Exercise 4

FIVE POSITIVE AND FIVE
NEGATIVE CHARACTERISTICS

Positive

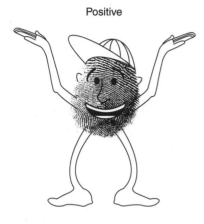

List Five Positive Characteristics

1._____

2._____

3._____

4._____

5._____

List Five Negative Characteristics

Negative

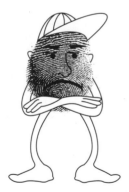

1._____

2._____

3._____

4._____

5._____

Endnotes

1. Virginia Satir, *Meditations and Inspirations* (Berkeley, CA: Celestial Arts, 1985), 17.

2. Mary Wilkes, and C. Bruce Crosswait, *Professional Development the Dynamics of Success* (San Diego: Harcourt Brace Jovanovich, Inc., 1991), 226-28.

3. Satir, *Meditations* 37.

Resources

1. Anderson, Mary Ann. *Nursing Leadership, Management and Professional Practice for the LPN, LVN*. Philadelphia: F. A. Davis Co., 1997.

2. Beattie, Melody. *Codependent No More: How to Stop Controlling Others and Start Caring for Yourself*. New York: Hazelton Information Education, 1996.

3. *Codependent No More: Beyond Codependency*. New York: Fine Communications, 1997.

4. Milliken, Mary Elizabeth. *Understanding Human Behavior: A Guide for Health Care Providers*. 6th ed. (Albany, NY: Delmar Publishers, 1998).

Chapter 2

Basic Communications Skills

Procedural Goal

To enhance the student's understanding and use of communication skills related to interpersonal relations in the medical office.

Learning Objectives

Upon completion of this unit, when given a written examination, the student will respond to the following with a minimum of ____% accuracy within the defined class period for the exam.

- List and define the four basic elements of the communication cycle.
- Identify or list the four modes or channels of communication most pertinent in our every day exchange.
- Analyze the five Cs of Communication and describe their communication effectiveness.
- Define the term *kinesics* and identify its communication effectiveness.
- Identify and explain the two keys to successful communication.
- Demonstrate nonverbal communication behaviors.

facial expression	touch
territoriality	position
posture	gestures/mannerisms

- List communication objectives to remember when conversing with diverse populations.
- Discuss the influence of technology on communication.
- Describe characteristics of the following management leaders:

  authoritarian

  participative

  MBWAs—Management by Wandering Around
- Describe a minimum of six roadblocks to communication and explain their affect on therapeutic communication.
- Identify three listening goals for the health professional.

When a young woman discovers she is pregnant, the news can be either joyous or devastating. For one young woman named Elaine it was not good news. She was unemployed, had no money, and was very much alone. Her desperation took her to the welfare office. Elaine realized she needed proper care for herself and the baby.

As time passed, she realized that she did not have what she wanted for her baby—a place to live, two loving parents, proper medical attention, and a mother who was emotionally mature and financially secure. Elaine chose adoption as the best solution. She finally selected an adoption agency after investigating several.

After several weeks and no opportunity to identify for the agency the kind of parents she would like for her baby, and little or no prenatal care assistance, she left the agency and decided to work through a private attorney for the adoption.

After only two conversations with the attorney who explained his services for birth mothers and adoptive parents, her self-esteem improved. She completed a detailed questionnaire describing herself and her family. She completed an equally detailed summary of the kind of qualities she was looking for in parents for her baby. The attorney insisted she receive prenatal care and provided her with the proper resources. Soon he matched her with a set of prospective parents.

Even though the decision had been made about who the adoptive parents would be prior to the baby's birth, Elaine knew the final separation would be very difficult. Elaine's obstetrician and his office staff knew of her decision. They described for her what the procedure would be in the hospital, and even arranged for her not to be in the maternity ward. But at no time, did they discourage her from seeing her baby or deny her any rights of any other expectant mother.

At the time of the baby's delivery, the reckoning came. The comments and the nonverbal actions of the hospital staff would make the difference. She was given the same treatment any other expectant mother would receive, and her best friend and baby coach were ushered into the delivery room with her. When the baby was born, the delivery room nurse asked Elaine if she wanted to hold the baby. When Elaine said no, the nurse held Elaine's hand, smiled, and told her that was fine. She could hold the baby, see the baby, even feed the baby at any time if she wanted.

Later that day, Elaine would appear at the nursery room window asking to see her baby. During the next twenty-four hours, while the attorney and adoptive parents were being notified, Elaine would hold, feed, and change this baby girl she was about to release. The adoptive parents had flown over fifteen hundred miles to receive the baby, so they were still a few hours away when it was time for Elaine to be discharged from the hospital.

Elaine and the adoptive parents had agreed that the baby should not go to a foster home for even a few moments, so the nurses made arrangements for Elaine to remain in the hospital, without additional charge, until the adoptive parents arrived.

The tearful exchange took place later and Elaine gave her daughter to be loved and cared for by the adoptive parents. One nurse assisted the ecstatic adoptive mother while another walked the birth mother through the hospital dismissal. Elaine was deeply saddened by her loss, but she was not broken or ashamed.

This story is repeated every day around the country. Can you see how it might be quite different if the comments and actions of the allied health professional were critical and judgmental? Can you cite examples of both social and therapeutic communications? A closer look at basic communication skills will help you assess therapeutic communications.

Communication Cycle

Communication is sending and receiving messages. Sometimes we are aware or conscious of the messages being sent or received and sometimes we are not. We are, however, always sending and receiving messages whether or not we are aware of them.

Communication is a compound action in which two or more people participate. As shown in Figure 2-1, there are four basic elements involved in the communication cycle: 1) a sender, 2) a message and the channel or mode of communication, 3) a receiver, and 4) feedback.

The Sender

The sender begins the communication cycle by creating or encoding the message. The sender must formulate a clear thought to send. There is great value in choosing words carefully in order to send a clear message to the receiver.

The Message

The message is the content to be communicated. The four channels or modes of communication most pertinent in our everyday exchange include: 1) speaking, 2) listening, 3) gestures or body language, and 4) writing. These may also be categorized into verbal and nonverbal communication.

How we send and how we perceive messages to a large extent is based on the influences suggested in Chapter 1.

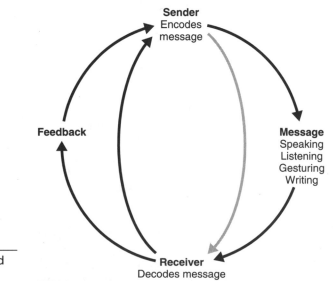

Figure 2-1

The communication cycle and channels of communication

Regardless of these influences, the message sent must be adapted to fit the situation and the receiver.

Recently a friend said to his wife, "I'm going to jump in the shower now." His two-and-a-half-year-old daughter overheard the comment. Several days later, she was found jumping in the shower. She understood his message in a very literal way. How and what we communicate is learned primarily by listening to and observing others. A two-and-a-half-year-old will interpret messages differently than an adult.

Each of these channels of communication has its appropriateness. In some instances, a written message may be the most effective means of communication. In other cases, spoken communication may be best.

The Receiver

A receiver is the recipient of the sender's message. The receiver must decode the message by evaluating the communication. The primary sensory skill used in verbal communication is listening. The spoken words, as well as the tone and pitch of voice, carry meaning. Any emphasis made by the sender must be fully understood by the receiver for the message to have meaning.

Feedback

Feedback occurs when the receiver and sender verify their perception of the message. Feedback may be either verbal or nonverbal. It reveals to the sender whether the message was interpreted accurately and enhances understanding by verifying and/or clarifying any misunderstanding.

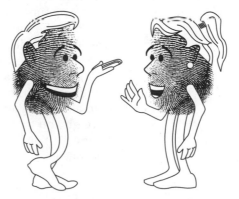

Sender and receiver must verify
their peceptions of the message.

Verbal Communications

When the message is spoken, we have verbal communication. Mere spoken words, however, carry no message unless the words have meaning. If you overhear a conversation in a language foreign to you, you are a witness to verbal communication, but you may not understand the message.

The spoken word, to have any meaning, must be understood by all parties to the communication. Mary Wilkes and C. Bruce Crosswait in their book *Professional Development* have identified the five Cs of communication in business. They are: 1) complete, 2) clear, 3) concise, 4) courteous, and 5) cohesive. These five Cs apply equally well to therapeutic communications.

The message must be *complete*, with all the necessary information given. It appears that the adoption agency first told Elaine she would be able to choose her baby's parents. What she discovered much later in the process was that she would not be able to do so until she had signed papers releasing the baby. The message was incomplete, even misleading, in its detail.

The information given in the message must also be *clear*. It must be spoken in terms understandable to both parties. It is best to enunciate carefully with good diction and keep objects out of and away from your mouth. Verbal communication will be most clear when there is eye contact.

A *concise* message is one that does not include unnecessary information. Imagine how different the message would have been had the delivery room nurse said to Elaine, "Well, you really should hold this baby. She is yours. I'd certainly hold her if she were mine."

A message must always be *courteous* if it is to be therapeutic. Any time communication is not considerate, there is a risk that the message will be unclear, even not received because of the defenses likely to be present in either the sender or the receiver.

A *cohesive* message is logical and in order. It does not jump abruptly from one subject to another. You would not say to a client, "Please remove all your clothes. No, we better weigh you first. Or do you want to give us a urine sample now?" You have confused the receiver and lost his attention.

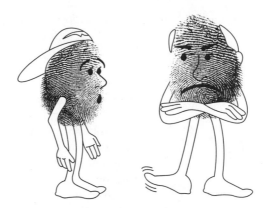

Nonverbal communication accounts
for about 70 percent of the message.

Nonverbal Communications

Taber's Cyclopedic Dictionary defines body language as the unconscious use of postures, gestures, or other forms of non-verbal expression in communication. **Kinesics** is defined as the systematic study of the body and the use of its static and dynamic position as a means of communication. Nonverbal communication does not involve speaking in words, but uses gestures and mannerisms. Nonverbal communication is the language we learn first. It is learned seemingly automatically as infants learn to smile in response to a smile or loving touches on the cheek long before they respond verbally. Much of our body language is a learned behavior and is greatly influenced by the culture in which we are raised.

Feelings are communicated quite well nonverbally. Since nonverbal communication is much less subject to conscious control, emotional dimensions are often expressed nonverbally. The body naturally expresses our true repressed feelings. Most of the negative messages we express nonverbally are unintended. But whether they are intentional or not, the message is relayed. Experts tell us that 70 percent of communication is nonverbal. The tone of voice communicates 23 percent of the message and only 7 percent of the message is actually communicated in what is said.

Two Key Points to Successful Communication

There are two key points to remember in successful communication. First, there must be congruency between the verbal and the nonverbal message. This means the two messages must be in agreement or be consistent with one another. If I verbally tell you I am not angry, but speak in angry tones, have my fists clinched and my face contorted, I am sending a mixed message. Chances are you will believe my nonverbal message rather than the verbal.

The second key to successful communication is to remember nonverbal cues appear in groups. The grouping of gestures, facial expressions, and postures into nonverbal statements is known as **clustering**. In the previous example, the tone of voice, the gestures of clinched fists, and facial expression form a nonverbal statement or cluster of cues to true feelings and emotions.

Facial Expression

Perhaps the most important nonverbal communicator is facial expression. It has been said that the eyes mirror the soul. The eyes communicate several kinds of messages. Have you ever seen laughter and joy in another's eyes? Have you seen grief or pain reflected in the eyes?

Eye contact is another form of facial expression and is often viewed as a sign of interest in the individual. It provides cues to indicate that what others say is important. A long stare may be interpreted as an invasion of privacy, which creates an uncomfortable, uneasy feeling. A lack of eye contact in Western culture is usually interpreted to mean a lack of involvement or avoidance.

Certain movements of the eyebrow seem to indicate questioning while others may disclose feelings of amusement, surprise, puzzlement, or worry. The manner in which the forehead is wrinkled also sends similar messages.

Touch

Touch is one of the most sensitive means of communication. Touch often is used to express deep feelings that are impossible to express verbally. Touch can be a very powerful means of communication as it expresses what cannot be expressed in words.

For all allied health professionals, many tasks involve touching the client. Most clients will understand and accept the touching behavior as it is related to the medical setting. Some clients, though, are not comfortable being touched, so sensitivity is essential. If you find yourself in a helping situation or profession and feel uncomfortable touching, self-analysis or awareness may be necessary.

Touch is often synonymous with reassurance, understanding, and caring. It is important to assess our level of comfort and that of the client in relation to the use of touch. When we are comfortable using touch and when we are sensitive to a client's level of acceptance to touch, we can use touch in a therapeutic manner.

Territoriality

Territoriality is the distance at which we are comfortable with others. It may be determined by sociocultural influences. We can think of it as the invisible fence used to keep a dog in the yard. No one can see it. However, the way in which we define our boundaries is evident to others.

We feel threatened when others invade our personal space without our consent. Examples of personal space are listed for your consideration.

Intimate — touching to $1\frac{1}{2}$ feet
Personal — $1\frac{1}{2}$ to 4 feet
Social — 4 to 12 feet
Public — 12 to 15 feet[1]

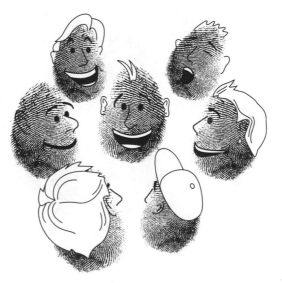

"Aren't you glad I showered this morning?"

Many cultures uphold these four categories of spatial relationships, however, the distances may vary from one culture to another.

Many medically related tasks involve invading another's personal space. It is beneficial to explain procedures that intrude another's space before beginning the procedure. This gives the client some control and a sense of dignity and worth.

Position

When speaking with a client, it is helpful to maintain a close but comfortable position. Standing over a client denotes superiority, while too much distance may be interpreted as being exclusive or avoiding. Movement toward a client usually indicates warmth, liking, interest, acceptance, and trust. Moving away may suggest dislike, disinterest, boredom, indifference, suspicion, or impatience (see Figure 2-2).

Figure 2-2

Positive posture and position encourage therapeutic communication. *(Courtesy of Carl Howard/Albany Medical Center)*

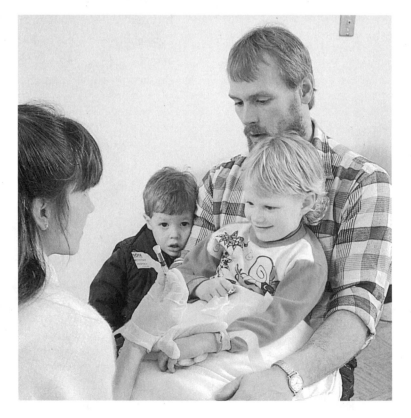

Posture

Like distance, posture is important to the allied health care professional. We tighten up in threatening situations and relax in a threatening environment. Posture may be used as a barometer for our feelings. For example, sitting with the limbs crossed sends a message of closure and avoidance; lying back in a chair with the arms up and hands clasped behind the head indicates an openness to suggestions.

Slumped shoulders may signal depression, discouragement, or in some cases even pain. It is important to validate the messages before continuing a procedure. For example, you may ask the client, " Are you comfortable?" or "Is this position too painful?" Technicians must be careful to be in tune to the client's physical discomfort.

Gestures/Mannerisms

Most of us use gestures or "talk" with our hands to some degree. Gestures are useful in emphasizing ideas, creating and holding others' attention, and in relieving stress.

Some common gestures and their meanings are:

Finger tapping – impatience, nervousness

Shrugged shoulders – indifference, discouragement

Rubbing the nose – puzzlement

Whitened knuckles and clenched fists – anger

Fidgeting – nervousness

It is important to recognize that nonverbal communication helps understanding and frequently is more powerful than verbal communication. It is also more enduring and has more persuasive power than verbal communication. We are more apt to read and believe the nonverbal message than the verbal message.

Word of Caution

It must be remembered, however, that nonverbal communication can easily be misinterpreted. The folded arms may mean the person is cold, not closed to communication. The wrinkled brow may indicate the person has a headache, not a questioning or doubting attitude. Look for congruency between verbal and nonverbal communication for a clear message.

In the illustration in this module's opening scenario, when the delivery room nurse asked Elaine if she would like to hold the baby, the verbal and nonverbal messages were congruent. When Elaine said no, the nurse held Elaine's hand, smiled, and told her that was fine. Together, the cluster of mannerisms used by the delivery room nurse said "I understand, I care, and your response is appropriate."

Communication with Diverse Populations

When communicating with diverse populations it is important to remember that meanings are given to different words based on the user's experiences, cultures, and ethnicity. Many translate the English they hear and see into their native language, process the information, and then translate it back into English. They have not yet learned to *think* in English. Therefore, when these populations seek medical treatment, there may be a hesitancy to freely discuss their problems or to ask questions regarding their health care or payment methods. Understanding various cultures and their values, beliefs, and mannerisms will greatly enhance the ability to communicate effectively.

The Asian population tends to be identified as Chinese, Japanese, Vietnamese, Cambodian, Hmong, Laotian, Korean, Philippino, Thai, Samoan, and Pacific Islanders of Asian descent. These cultures are relative newcomers to the United States fighting to reverse a variety of prejudices thrust upon them. This population believes that strength and support come from the family and community and not from and outside source. Therefore, Asians are more hesitant to approach non-Asians for assistance.

Individuals who represent the Spanish background may include Chicano, Latino, Hispanic, Mexican-American, Puerto Rican, persons with a Spanish surname, and persons of Spanish extraction. This broad ethnicity represents varied communication styles throughout the country. Family and interpersonal relationships between persons are of the highest value to this population. Trust levels must be established and maintained and care should be taken to not be seen as "savior."

Among the native American Indian population, there are more than 700 different cultures. The highest value of this group is oneness with the Great Spirit. Eye contact during conversation varies from tribe to tribe, but generally speaking, touching someone during casual conversation is considered unacceptable. Emotions are not typically displayed or expressed and verbal communication is usually brief.

The Federal government defines Pacific Islanders based on a geographic location. Many of this culture believe that knowledge is finite, meaning that there is only a limited amount of knowledge. Often they feel that knowledge shared, is knowledge lost, and only the chiefs and the priests are allowed to be educated. Few of the native dialects exist in written form, and age and position rather than education govern positions of respect and authority. Many Pacific Island cultures consider it inappropriate for an individual to take pride in a personal achievement and only that which enhances the community is recognized and honored.

Racial prejudices and discrimination issues continue to be of concern to the African-American population. These issues are beginning to be dispelled with increasing numbers of black role models in positions of respect and authority.

In general, Eastern cultures believe silence indicates respect and trust and that the spoken word pollutes the exchange. These cultures place emphasis on heart-to-heart communication that implies that people can intuitively grasp the meaning of the message. With these thoughts in mind, Westerners must listen more and talk less.

Gestures and mannerisms may have different meanings based on culture. It is important to understand the cultures with which we communicate and listen carefully, and not jump to conclusions based on our own culture and belief. Recognize, also, that individuals within a particular culture unite and support each other in conflict or crisis.

Influence of Technology on Communication

Face-to-face communication, telephone conversations, paper memos are being replaced with e-mail, faxes, and telecommunication conferences in today's technological office. We use cellular phones and laptop computers linked to a network of computers that communicate with satellite offices which are linked to corporate headquarters which may be in another part of the community or even in another country.

In the future we may need to reevaluate the communication interactions required to function and advance in the interactive technological office environment. The content of the message will be examined for credibility rather than one's dress, eye contact, facial expression, vocal inflection, and posture. Computer-mediated communication and a greater reliance on cyberspace technology will greatly impact communication in the twenty-first century.

Team Communication

In order to communicate effectively as a team member, we must take time to develop skills that will ensure levels of trust and to build into the team a sense of worth and importance. Consideration also must be given to cultural diversity and to understanding ways in which other cultures communicate. For example, during a business meeting, Americans prefer to be seated either face-to-face or at right angles to each other. Asian cultures prefer side-by-side positions. Americans generally follow Maslow's Hierarchy of Needs (refer to page 120) with self-actualization as the pinnacle whereas the Asian society emphasize belonging.

Authoritarian leaders often use a domineering and direct communication style when managing personnel. **Participative** leaders on the other hand elicit suggestions from subordinates and encourage open discussion. Another form of leadership is **management by wandering around (MBWA)**. These leaders interact with those they supervise to reward positive performance and discourage negative behavior in a manner that reinforces rather than diminishes self-esteem.

Listening Skills

Listening is often identified as the passive portion of communication. However, if done well, listening is very active. Good listeners have their eyes upon the speaker, are attentive, and are aware of the nonverbal messages as well as the verbal information coming from the sender. Effective listening requires concentration.

Therapeutic listening includes listening with a "third ear," that is, being aware of what the client is *not* saying or picking up on hints to the real message. In the scenario of Mrs. Nelson at the beginning of this section, her primary care physician was either unaware of the nonverbal cues and hints being made or chose to see them as unimportant.

The health professional should have three listening goals: (1) to improve listening skills sufficiently so that clients are heard accurately, (2) either to listen for what is not being said or for information transmitted only by hints, and (3) to determine how accurately the message has been received.

A technique that has been used by many and is suggested by professionals is the ability to paraphrase the client's message or statement. This technique allows the receiver of the message to return the message to the sender, perhaps worded differently, allowing the sender to acknowledge the accuracy of the message.

Sender:	"Will I be able to use my medical coupons for prenatal care in your clinic?"
Receiver:	"You're concerned about whether our doctor accepts medical coupons for payment."
Sender:	"That's correct. I have no money. My baby will be adopted, but I know we need proper medical care."
Receiver:	"Our office does take medical coupons and you will receive the best of care. Would you like to make an appointment?"

This example shows both active listening and therapeutic communication skills. The office assistant heard both concerns—the monetary concern and the concern for proper care.

Health professionals must be prudent in how they use active listening techniques, however. It is not appropriate to paraphrase everything the client says, otherwise the client begins to feel stupid or believes the professional has a hearing problem.

One of the greatest barriers to listening occurs when receivers find themselves thinking about something else or themselves while they are trying to listen. It does not work well to try to concentrate on the other person if your mind keeps flipping back to yourself. When this happens, it is best to pull concentration back to the sender, apologize if necessary, and get on with the communication.

LISTEN

When I ask you to listen to me
    and you start giving advice
    you have not done what I asked.

When I ask you to listen to me
    and you begin to tell me why I shouldn't feel that way,
    you are trampling on my *feelings*.

When I ask you to listen to me
    and you feel you have *to do* something to solve my problem,
    you have failed me, strange as that may seem.

Listen! All I asked, was that you listen.
    not talk or do—just hear me.
Advice is cheap: 10 cents will get you both Dear Abby and
    Billy Graham in the same newspaper.
And I can do for myself; I'm not helpless.
    Maybe discouraged and faltering, but not helpless.

When you do something for me *that I can and need to do*
    for myself, you contribute to my fear and weakness.
But, when you accept as a simple fact that I do feel what I feel,
    no matter how irrational, then I can quit trying to convince
    you and can get about the business of understanding what's
    behind this irrational feeling.
    And when that's clear, the answers are obvious and I don't
    need advice.
Irrational feelings make sense when we understand what's behind
them.

Perhaps that's why prayer works, sometimes, for some people
    because God is mute, and he doesn't give advice or
    try to fix things. "They" just listen and let you work it out for
    yourself.

So, please listen and just hear me. And, if you want to
    talk, wait a minute for your turn; and I'll listen to you.

Anonymous[2]

Perhaps this bit of poetry so filled with wisdom is all that is necessary as a reminder that there is a time in communication, in listening, when silence is appropriate. So many times health professionals try to "fix" everything with a recommendation, a prescription, even advice. Sometimes, none of those things is necessary. The client simply needs someone to listen, to acknowledge the difficulty, and to remember that the client is not helpless in finding a solution to the problem.

Skill in communication takes years of practice and frequent review. It will never become perfect; we can only hope that we will become better at it each passing day. Communication is and always will be the very basis for any therapeutic relationship.

Exercise 1

To assist in assessing your level of comfort with territoriality and personal space, ask yourself the following questions.

1. How do I define my personal space?

2. Do I sit in the same classroom seat each day?

3. Do I have books or papers on my boundary lines?

4. Did I move someone else's paperwork that was encroaching upon my personal space?

5. Do I send subtle messages to others who may invade my territory unknowingly?

6. Do I take my half of the bed out of the middle?

7. Are you more comfortable with face-to-face communication or with "on-line" communication?

8. When seated in public transportation or at the theater, do I choose a personal space that is intimate (touching to $1\frac{1}{2}$ feet) or personal ($1\frac{1}{2}$ to 4 feet)? Does my personal space vary depending upon who I am with at the time?

9. When shopping at a mall, how close do I walk to others?

10. When I am in an elevator with a stranger, do I follow the social or public space differentiation?

11. How comfortable do I feel in multicultural groups?

12. When I am walking down the street, do I glance away or look the oncomer in the eye?

Exercise 2

Watch a thirty-minute television program with the volume off. If a VCR is available; record the program also. On a piece of paper, note and list the types of nonverbal communication used during the program.

Now that the program is over, evaluate the nonverbal cues observed to determine your understanding of the program content. Were the cues effective as communicators of the message? Do you have a good understanding of the message content or are you able to relate only to the emotional aspects of the communication?

If you recorded the program, take time to view it again with the volume **on**. Compare your understanding of the program content now with what you learned with the volume **off**.

Write a paragraph describing what you discovered during this exercise. Be certain to respond to the three points.

Exercise 3

Write a paragraph discussing a recent incident, preferably personal, in which a communicator failed to communicate what was intended. Analyze why this happened and how it could have been avoided.

Endnotes

1. Julius Fast, *Body Language* (New York: M. Evans and Company, Inc., 1970), 30-34.

2. David S. Bailey and Sharon O. Dreyer, *Therapeutic Approaches to the Care of the Mentally Ill* (Philadelphia: F. A. Davis Company Publishers, 1977), vi.

Resources

1. Chapman, Elwood N. *Your Attitude is Showing, A Primer of Human Relations*, 8th ed. (Upper Saddle River, NJ: Prentice-Hall Inc., 1996).

2. Fruehling, Rosemary, and Neil B. Oldham. *Working at Human Relations.* Eden Prairie, MN: Paradigm Press International, 1991.

3. Gamble, Teri Kwal, and Michael W. Gamble. *Contacts Communicating Interpersonally.* Needham Heights, MA: Allyn and Bacon, 1998.

4. Jarrow, Jane. "Serving Multiculturally Diverse Populations in Trio Programs: A Beginner's Guide from WESTOP." Conference report from Honolulu: 1990.

5. Lehmann, Helm. *Driver's Ed for Today's Managers.* Auburn, WA: Organizational Performance and Planning Institute, 1998.

6. Milliken, Mary Elizabeth. *Understanding Human Behavior*, 6th ed. (Albany, NY: Delmar Publishers, 1998).

7. Satir, Virginia. *Meditations and Inspirations.* Berkeley, CA: Celestial Arts, 1986.

8. Wilkes, Mary, and C. Bruce Crosswait. *Professional Development and the Dynamics of Success.* New York: Harcourt Brace Jovanovich Publishers, 1991.

Chapter 3

The Helping Interview

Procedural Goal

To enhance the student's understanding and use of communication skills related to interpersonal relations during the helping interview.

Learning Objectives

Upon completion of this unit, when given a written examination, the student will respond to the following with a minimum of _____% accuracy within the defined class period for the exam.

- Define *helping interview* and list the three primary components of the helping interview.
- List and contrast the feelings experienced by the individual giving help and the individual needing help.
- Identify a minimum of ten important preparations to be made by the helping professional before the interview takes place.
- Describe the following attributes and their use in the helping interview.

  risk/trust

  warmth/caring

  genuineness

sympathy/empathy

sincerity

- Describe the following responding skills and their use.

sharing observations

acknowledging feelings

clarifying and validating

reflecting and paraphrasing

- Discuss the *levels of need* and relate them to the helping interview.
- Define the following and differentiate how they encourage or discourage the therapeutic exchange.

closed questions

open questions

indirect statements

- Describe the following blocks to therapeutic communication.

reassuring clichés/stereotypical comments

giving advice/approval

requesting/requiring an explanation

belittling

defending

changing the subject/shifting

- Demonstrate or list the steps involved in an appropriate closure of a helping interview.

Interview Components

A helping interview is a conversation between a helping professional and a person in need and is a common tool of communications in any health care setting. Three components of the helping interview are:

1. The *orientation* of the professional and the client to each other
2. The *identification* of the client's problem
3. The resolution of the client's problem

The helping interview is usually planned for a set time and place and with the helping professional in control.

Control Factor

Control is a critical factor in the helping interview, but should not be abused. Even the use of the word patient implies a superior/inferior, higher/lower, more-knowledge/less-knowledge relationship. The helping interview clearly involves people in an unequal partnership. Being in a state of need or helplessness is not empowering. Consider the following feelings likely to describe giving and needing help.

Giving Help	Needing Help
Feeling important	Feeling unimportant or inadequate
Feeling useful	Feeling useless or depressed
Feeling powerful	Feeling powerless
Feeling gratified	Feeling frightened or embarrassed
Feeling happy	Feeling sad or angry

It is more pleasant to give help than to need help. Helping professionals must be constantly aware of how their status affects persons seeking help. Clients should be empowered as much as possible by the experience in the helping interview, since empowered clients are likely to participate more fully in their care and return to health faster (Figure 3-1).

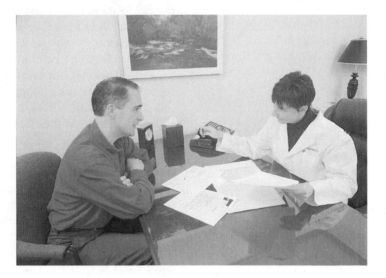

Figure 3-1

"Give clients as much dignity and empowerment as possible." *Comprehensive Medical Assisting Administrative & Clinical Competencies*, W. Lindh, M. Pooler, C. Tamparo, J. Cerrato, Delmar Publishers, Albany NY 1998.

Orientation

There are some important preparations to be made by the helping professional even before the interview takes place. Personal appearance and the appearance of the medical office or examination room are vital keys to getting the helping interview off to a good start.

Your personal appearance must be professional and your grooming impeccable. The health professional, always alert to the control of any disease-producing organisms, will remember that personal cleanliness helps to reduce the number of pathogens and inhibits their transmission. A daily bath, an effective deodorant, and fresh breath are essential personal characteristics. Hair that is clean, off the collar, and out of the face is both sanitary and easy to care for. Even the most attractive hair should not be on the collar while at work. Nails should be trimmed and neatly manicured. Any polish worn should only be clear. Hands must be washed between clients. Your uniform should fit properly and be appropriate to the setting. Any aftershave or cologne must be very light or omitted completely. It is best to wear no jewelry with the exception of post earrings and wedding rings. A name tag that includes your title is most helpful.

Do not be fooled by some who will tell you that such careful detail to this professional dress is unimportant. Quite the opposite is true. The client expects that you are professional, that you dress the part. In fact, the client may have difficulty trusting someone who is too casual in appearance.

If the client is to come to your office or you are to go to the examination room, consider those surroundings. Will the setting encourage an equal relationship? Are you seated near the client or with a desk between you? Is the examination room so small that the client must sit on the table? If possible, be seated facing the client and at the same level. It is better to never have the client disrobed during the orientation phase of the interview.

Greet your client in a pleasant manner and with a name when possible. Introduce yourself and give your title if the client may not know it. Be certain to get the client's name and pronounce it correctly. Do not address the client informally unless the client requests that you do so. If the interview is conducted in the examination room, knock before entering.

Be aware of your tone and voice volume. Do not speak in a monotone. Make certain the client hears and understands you. If there is a language barrier or speech problem, get an expert to help you. You sound and appear silly if you try to speak a language in which you really have only a little knowledge. Time is an important element. The health professional must have time to hear the client. The helping interview is no place for there to be a chance for misunderstanding.

Risk/Trust

As the interview gets underway, the conversation involves a fair amount of risk on the part of the client. There is the need for the helping professional to build an atmosphere of trust making the risk easier. As the trust level increases, it is easier for the client to share feelings and attitudes about the problem. Trust has to be earned. Without it, the helping relationship will go no further than mere introductions. The helping professional is responsible for nurturing mutual trust.

Warmth/Caring

Warmth may be defined as an attitude expressing caring and concern. It is primarily communicated through facial expressions, such as a caring look or smile that crosses all cultural differences. A gentle touch or a calm, reassuring voice also expresses warmth and caring. This attitude is helpful in creating a nonthreatening atmosphere in which the client feels free to express concerns. Caring expresses a liking or regard for others and communicates a watchfulness for cues that may indicate the problem and its possible solution.

Genuineness

Genuineness is being real and honest with others. The health care professional must be able to communicate honestly with others while being careful not to blame or condemn. Genuineness assures there will be congruency between the verbal and nonverbal messages. Genuineness and acceptance are partners in the helping interview.

Sympathy/Empathy

To show sympathy is to respond to the emotional state of others and to acknowledge the feelings expressed by clients. Sympathy states "I am available to you." Empathy is the ability to accept another's private world as if it were your own. It is fair and sensitive; it is an awareness of others' situations and what they are experiencing. It communicates identification with and understanding of another's situation. Empathy states "I'm available to walk this road with you."

Sincerity

Sincerity involves those attributes already identified as well as creating an atmosphere that is free from hypocrisy. The health care professional who is sincere is forthright, candid, and truthful. Health care professionals must be sincere in their intentions and communications with others.

Identification of Problem

Once the orientation phase has been completed and the trust level is fairly established, it is time to turn attention to the problem or problems that are shared by the client. As well as keeping in mind that you must listen with the "third ear," there are a number of techniques that will ease the communication between clients and health professionals. These techniques may be referred to as *responding skills* and are identified in the next section.

Sharing Observations

Observations will focus on both the client's physical and emotional state. The statement "You seem upset" conveys concern and interest in knowing more and comes from the health professional's observation of the client. The tone of voice, eye contact, and body position are all factors to be considered in observations. Statements such as "You are trembling" or "You seem to be in pain" are examples of shared observations. Such statements encourage the client to continue.

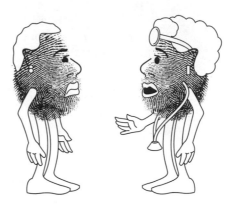

"You seem to be in pain."

Acknowledging Feelings

Sharing observations is a way to acknowledge the client's feelings. This responding skill communicates to clients that their feelings are understood and accepted. It encourages verbalization by providing a safe, nonthreatening environment. An example of such an acknowledgment is "I see you are worried by the pain you're having." Such acknowledgment makes it easier for clients to reveal their symptoms.

Clarifying and Validating

Clarifying is used when the health professional is not certain of the meaning of the message communicated. Such statements as "I'm not sure I understand what you mean." or "Do you mean...?" are examples of clarification. Words used during an exchange may hold different meanings to others, so clarifying is important. This is especially critical when languages are different or may be easily misunderstood. For the message to be therapeutic, both parties must have the same meaning and use the terms in the same manner.

Reflecting and Paraphrasing

Reflecting focuses on the emotional aspect of the client's expression. It involves listening to the verbal message as well as considering the nonverbal cues being sent. The facial expression and tone of voice will provide insight regarding the meaning of the message and its congruency. When using reflecting skills, "You feel" will often be used at the beginning or within the response; for example, "You feel like the medicine is not helping."

Paraphrasing simply restates in the professional's own words what the client said. Its focus is more on the cognitive aspects of the message than on the feeling. Paraphrasing allows the client to hear what was just said and to verify the accuracy of the professional's listening ability. It is often helpful to tie together reflecting and paraphrasing. Using words such as "you feel...because..." connects the two skills easily; for example, "You feel the medicine is not helping because you still have the headaches."

Levels of Need

Paul Welter, in *How to Help a Friend*[1], identifies the helping relationship and levels of need. To become an effective helper, it is necessary to recognize what level of need your client has. Although this chart was established for helping friends, much of it can be adapted to recognizing the needs of clients who come for help. See Table 3-1, Levels of Need.

Recognizing that clients have different levels of need helps professionals to focus attention correctly. Keeping in mind the attributes identified and the levels of need creates an atmosphere in which questions can be asked that will assist clients to fully identify the problems they face.

Questioning Techniques

There is real skill in knowing how to ask questions in a manner that helps the client express problems. These questions and answers are important to the identification and resolution of the problem. Also, they become the foundation for the client's medical record. There are three major types of questions useful during the helping interview, and each has its appropriateness.

Table 3-1 Levels of Need

Level and Definition	Characteristics of Person in Need	Effective Helping Response
Problem Has a solution.	Asks specific question; wants immediate advice or information.	Supply information or advice.
Predicament No easy solution.	Often feels trapped; is not helped by advice.	The helper gets involved; works for openness.
Crisis A very large predicament; short-term.	Has a sense of urgency; may both want and not want help.	Expects you to help; bring client into present; accept emotions.
Panic A state of fear; sees only one way out.	Does not listen; mind is caught in dreadful future event; nonrational.	Move client from panic to "hold"; use touch; eye contact.
Shock A numbed or dazed condition.	Fails to take action; mind lapses for short time; unable to recall lapse.	Must act for this person. Stay with this person until back to normal.

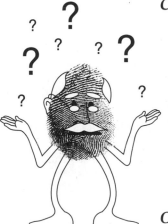

Closed Questions

Closed questions are useful in collecting information during the client history and are most common at the beginning of the verbal exchange. They do not require the individual being asked the question to enlarge upon the answer. The questions usually begin with *do*, *is*, or *are*, and are answered with a simple yes, no, or a brief phrase. Examples of closed questions are:

> "Are you experiencing pain now?"
> "Do you feel pain when raising your arm?"
> "Is the bandage too tight?"

Open-Ended Questions

Open-ended questions are most helpful for therapeutic communication because they encourage clients to identify more of the problem. They do not put words into clients' mouths, rather they allow clients to express their own thoughts and feelings. Open-ended questions usually begin with *how*, *what*, or *could*. They are an invitation for clients to express more detail. Examples of open-ended questions are:

> "Could your new job be responsible for a change in your eating habits?"
> "How did you sleep last night?"
> "What did the doctor tell you about this medication?"

Indirect Statements

Open-ended questions can be reworded so that they become indirect statements. Indirect statements call for a response from the client, but do not make the client feel like he/she is being questioned. They do, however, encourage verbalization and express interest in the client from the helping professional. Examples of indirect statements are:

> "I'd like to hear about your new therapy program."
> "Tell me about your fears."

During the helping interview, it is beneficial to stay away from the use of questions that begin with *why*. When questions begin with *why*, clients often become defensive or feel they are being accused. Questions beginning with *how* or *what* are much more effective. This and other blocks to communication are identified in the next section.

Roadblocks to Communication

There are so many roadblocks to communication that one marvels at how any communication is effective. In therapeutic communication, preventing roadblocks is vital to a quality relationship with the client.

Some of the most common roadblocks to therapeutic communications are:

> reassuring clichés
> giving advice/approval
> requiring explanations
> belittling/contradicting/criticizing
> defending
> changing subject/shifting
> moralizing/lecturing
> shaming/threatening

Health care professionals must keep in mind that when clients seek care for some problem or ailment, they have psychological and mental attitudes that are delicate and must be handled with care to put the client at ease. Therefore, paying close attention to communication roadblocks is vital.

Reassuring Clichés

Reassuring **clichés** are often given automatically and consist of patterned responses, trite expressions, or empty, meaningless phrases. When the health professional senses the client may be anxious or stressed, reassuring clichés may be expressed in an effort to reduce these feelings. Although the health professional may use these terms in an effort to reduce the client's concerns, the client may interpret them to mean the professional does not understand the problem or is not interested in becoming involved. These phrases may also be used by health professionals to reduce their own personal anxieties. Examples of reassuring clichés are:

> "Everything will be all right."
> "You don't need to worry about that."
> "Keep your chin up. Hang in there."

Giving Advice/Approval

Giving advice may occur when health professionals act from a subconscious effort to have all the answers or feel the need to control the client's thoughts or actions. When we tell clients what they should do, we impose our opinions and solutions on them. This advice-giving usually begins with "If I were you..." or "You should..." Recognition of the fact that these phrases are being used should trigger a warning signal to stop. We can never be in the exact circumstances or situations of another person. Remember, the goal is to sufficiently empower the client who will then be able to recognize what advice might be needed. Even when the physician gives directions to clients, the phrase can be "My recommendation is..."

Requiring Explanations

Asking clients to explain their reasons for feelings, behaviors, or thoughts requires them to analyze and explain these experiences. Questions that ask *Why* are intimidating. Examples are, "Why do you think you are feeling that way?" and

"Why did you do that?" Often clients may not understand the reasons for the discomfort to begin with. They may understand the discomfort but not know how to describe it or may not have sufficient trust in the professional to risk sharing their feelings. During the helping interview, health professionals should ask clients to describe their feelings rather than explain them. This approach is nonthreatening and communicates to clients that their feelings are acceptable. It encourages clients to continue describing their situation.

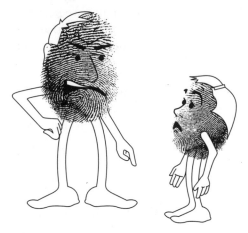

"You shouldn't feel that way."

Belittling/Contradicting/Criticizing

Expressions such as "You couldn't have bled that much" or "You shouldn't feel that way" send a message to the client that "You are mistaken; your feelings are unimportant." When a client comes with a concern or a complaint, responding negatively will close the communication process immediately. The client feels what the client feels. Even if you, the professional, know that what is being described is impossible, clients are still the only ones who know their own body and feelings. Listen and acknowledge the client's statements. Do not contradict.

There is never any time in a therapeutic relationship to criticize clients. Even if a client does something that is foolish, harmful, and extremely unhealthy, criticism does not open the line of communication for wise, safe, and healthy advice or information.

Defending

"No one in this clinic would tell you that." When the health professional defends something or someone the client has criticized, it implies the client has no right to express feelings, concerns, or impressions. This contradiction will block the therapeutic exchange and prevent further verbalization by the client.

Changing the Subject/Shifting

When the health professional changes the subject or shifts to new topics, the direction of the conversation will be controlled by the professional rather than allowing clients to discuss freely what they choose. Shifting the trust of the helping interview toward the health professional's perceptions also blocks the exchange. Once the client has been blocked, he/she may discontinue future attempts to share feelings, concerns, or problems. Examples of changing the subject or shifting are:

Client: "I'd like to die."

Professional: "Did your daughter visit this week?"

The professional might change the subject because he/she is uncomfortable with the topic or simply may want to gain information related to another specific subject. Care should be used in changing the subject or shifting to a new topic to be certain it is appropriate to the present verbal exchange.

Moralizing/Lecturing

Health professionals who easily criticize probably moralize also. Even though the client appears with a condition caused by a lifestyle that is totally contrary to both society standards and yours, expressing your judgment is unlikely to have a positive effect on the client. When you moralize, you are unable to fully and completely accept the client's needs. In Elaine's situation, her self-esteem was partly preserved by the refusal of her health care professionals to moralize over her decision. Health professionals who work daily with substance-abuse addicts must not moralize, but be able to see the person who was or who can be again.

Health professionals, with all their knowledge and many years of experience are apt to lecture. They might feel the lecture is quite appropriate to the situation. Even when the sharing of information is vital to the client's well-being, to lecture only makes the client feel defensive or of little value.

Shaming/Threatening

To ridicule or shame a client will close communication immediately. Most often, this ridicule or shame is in the form of nonverbal rather than verbal communication. Health professionals have been taught not to ridicule or shame, but it often shows in actions rather than words. To laugh at a client's description of an ailment or misunderstanding of basic body functions is a common example of ridicule. To threaten a client with the consequences of some act only causes fear, submission, and resentment. It does nothing to encourage the client to change behavior. Clients are able to determine for themselves if their actions are damaging and what the consequences will be. Health care professionals who threaten are usually insecure or feel total responsibility for their clients. Neither characteristic is healthy.

Resolution of the Problem

As the helping interview comes to a close, it is hoped that some resolution of the problem is also obvious. While many problems will require ongoing care, there should be some problem resolution in each helping interview. It is important for the helping professional to use the clearest and most simple language since most clients have little or no knowledge of medical terminology. It is important to remember if the receiver has not understood the message as it was sent, no communication has taken place.

Most clients are seeking an explanation for their problem, want to know how resolution of the problem is going to affect their lives, how much time to allow for this resolution, and what future impact the problem may have. For example, a client who has been diagnosed with ulcerative colitis might be told: "Mr. Olson, the results of all our tests show that you have ulcerative colitis. We do not understand the cause of this illness, but there are no indications to believe that any serious damage has occurred at this time. With proper treatment and medication, we should be able to keep active flare-ups at a minimum and prevent further complications."

The interview might continue at this point into a discussion of the client's lifestyle. Continue the discussion with ways to help the client cope with the impact of this disease and a description of the treatment necessary. It might also continue as follows: "There is no cure for this disease and you may have many exacerbations and remissions throughout your life, but if this treatment works, there should be no complicating medical problems. However, it is important for us to treat this problem now, because untreated, it can become serious. It is a good idea for you to include more bulk and bran in your diet. I have a suggested nutritional plan here for you to consider. If certain foods cause diarrhea, then eliminate them from your diet or do not eat them during an active flare-up. In the active stage of this disease, avoid excess stress as much as possible. Also, I have a prescription to give you to assist the healing process in your lower colon and medication to help prevent complications. You should see an improvement in just several days."

Allow time for the client to think about what has just been said and to formulate any questions that have arisen. This is a good time to fill out the prescription or to get the nutritional guidelines from your file. Even saying "You must have some questions now, too" can be helpful to the client. If there are no questions at this point, remind the client: "Remember to call me any time you have a question. If you have any concerns or you are not better in a few days, call me. I will want to see you again in six weeks to make certain that we are on the right track."

It is most helpful to write instructions for clients or to provide them with some written material explaining the procedures they are to follow. The best medical advice can be lost if clients do not correctly follow instructions.

———

It cannot be emphasized enough that the helping interview will either be the key to a helping professional's success or the end of what might be a therapeutic relationship. Recall the incident identified at the beginning of this section with Mrs. Nelson who had been seriously injured by the dog. Consider how different the outcome might have been had her primary care physician been more "in tune" during the interview.

When Mrs. Nelson called her primary care physician, it would have been much more therapeutic had the assistant said, "Oh, Mrs. Nelson, how awful. You say the emergency room physician asked that you have a blood test this morning and that you have his records with you? We usually only see patients receiving complete physicals in the morning, but I believe that the doctor will want to comply with the emergency room physician. Would you mind if you had to wait a bit when you come in?"

Mrs. Nelson, who has already shown that she is a compliant client, responds in the affirmative and the assistant selects a time where the wait will be as minimal as possible. When she is ushered into the examination room with her physician and the blood has been taken, the doctor might have said, "My assistant tells me you had a frightening experience with a dog, Mrs. Nelson. Tell me what happened."

While the doctor listens and observes Mrs. Nelson, he will notice her bandaged head and finger and how uncomfortable she appears. It is likely that questions will be asked of Mrs. Nelson regarding the medical chart from the emergency room to further enhance the record. It seems important, also, for the doctor to say, "May I remove your bandage to have a look at your injury while the assistant is checking your blood count for us?"

Both head and finger wounds are examined and appropriately bandaged by the doctor. Through this process and a discussion of the fractured tailbone and ways to be more comfortable, Mrs. Nelson is still showing anxiety. The doctor might then say,

"You seem quite anxious and worried, Mrs. Nelson."

"Well, I am I guess. This is a heck of a spot to be in. I love dogs so much; to think I could be attacked by one! If I lose my little poodle, I will be really mad. And you know, we are about to celebrate our fifty-second wedding anniversary. We usually go someplace. I guess I won't be doing that, will I?"

"It is pretty hard to see a dog attack your dog and get hurt in the meantime, I know. I have a dog, and I think I would feel awful if something like that happened to her, especially when she did nothing to provoke the attack. How is your poodle?"

"Well, the vet says he will make it, but he looks awful. My husband picked him up at the vet this morning."

"As for going somewhere, you should still be able to go. You can remove this bandage tomorrow and come back in two days so I can remove the stitches. Then get yourself to the beauty shop and they will be able to cover up the part of your head they shaved. Your finger can be put into a more comfortable splint in a couple of days, too. The fractured tailbone is going to cause you the most problem for awhile, so it might be good to get away where you won't have the responsibilities of all your household chores. Let someone else do all your cooking and cleaning. Traveling with a comfortable pillow to sit on is the only suggestion I might make to you."

"But what in the world will I do in the meantime? Look at all the dried blood still matted in my hair. This is awful."

"My assistant will be able to get a lot of that out for you. She can get most of it; the rest will have to wait until the stitches are removed. Then you can have it shampooed."

"What a relief that would be. Maybe we still can take a little trip. Maybe even our poodle will be well enough to be gone for awhile, too. I'm certain I'll need some information from you for the dog owner's insurance. Will I be able to get that?"

"You call me and I'll be glad to supply anything that is required. Let me know if you have any problems with your injuries. I see that you are scheduled for your annual physical soon. Let's set that appointment for the first part of next month so we can check everything again for you."

Mrs. Nelson left the clinic with her hair a little cleaner, reassurances from her physician, recognition of the trauma she had been through, and another appointment. The therapeutic relationship will continue.

Exercise 1

If you agree with the authors that the noun "patient" implies an unequal partnership, what other nouns might you suggest to make the relationship more equal? What terms are common to other settings in an unequal partnership? Can you feel comfortable in using them? How do you feel about the use of the word client?

Exercise 2

Trust Walk

With a classmate or a friend, take a ten-minute walk around campus, your workplace, or your neighborhood. During the ten minutes, you must be blindfolded for five minutes while you rely on your partner to guide you and lead you. After the five minutes, exchange places with your partner who will then be blindfolded and led around by you.

Describe your feelings. Were you most comfortable as the leader or the follower? Why? Share your observations with the class. What does this exercise tell you about a client's level of risk and trust?

Exercise 3

With a classmate, practice your responding skills. Recall a time when you received treatment in a health care setting. One of you will play the role of the client, the other the role of the helping professional.

List shared observations, acknowledged feelings, examples of clarifying and validating, and reflecting or paraphrasing. Now switch roles. Repeat the exercise. You will observe how much easier it is the second time.

Exercise 4

Consider what your response might be for the following client statements.

1. "How come you sent me this bill? I don't owe you any money!"

   Response _____

2. Phone conversation: "These little green pills make me sick. I'm not going to take them any more."

   Response _____

3. "You told me Medicare would cover this."

   Response _____

4. "If you won't take medical coupons, who will?"

   Response _____

5. "You're not going to have to give little Johnnie a shot, are you?"

   Response _____

6. "Why won't you tell me the test results? Why do I have to talk to the doctor?"

   Response _____

Exercise 5

Journal Exercises

1. Keep a journal for a week. In this journal be aware of your friends and family members who might have a problem. Can you identify the levels of need? How about your own problems? Can you identify the levels of need and the helping responses?

2. Be aware of roadblocks to communications that you make or that you observe in other conversations. Make a note of these in your journal and identify how the roadblock could be changed to a helping response.

To be successful in these exercises, you will probably need to review daily the material in this unit that identifies levels of need and roadblocks.

Exercise 6

Identify the following as closed or open-ended questions, indirect statements, or roadblocks.

1. _____ How are you feeling today?

2. _____ You're looking pretty chipper today.

3. _____ Why did you do that?

4. _____ When I lift your leg, does it hurt?

5. _____ Oh, don't worry; everything will be fine.

6. _____ You're not getting old.

7. _____ Oh, it couldn't possibly feel like that.

8. _____ You say the accident happened this morning?

9. _____ What did the doctor tell you about the test results?

10. _____ Tell me about the test results.

11. _____ Could you tell me when you think this started?

12. _____ I'd like to hear about your new job.

13. _____ Why do you think you feel this way?

Endnote

1. Paul Welter, *How to Help a Friend* (Wheaton, IL: Tyndale House Publishing, 1990).

Resources

1. Anderson, Mary Ann. *Nursing Leadership, Management and Professional Practice for the LPN, LVN*. Philadelphia: F. A. Davis Company, 1997.
2. Davis, Edwin. *Customer Relations for Careers*. Westerville, OH: McGraw Hill, 1991.
3. Chapman, Elwood N. *Your Attitude is Showing, A Primer of Human Relations*, 8th ed. (Upper Saddle River, NJ. Prentice-Hall, Inc., 1996).

Chapter 4

Defense Mechanisms

Procedural Goal

To enhance the student's awareness of defense mechanisms and aid in understanding when they can be helpful or harmful.

Learning Objectives

Upon completion of this unit, when given a written examination, the student will respond to the following with a minimum of_____% accuracy within the defined class period for the exam.

- Define the term *defense mechanism* and understand when defense mechanisms may be helpful or harmful.
- Describe the following defense mechanisms:

regression	repression
sublimination	rationalization
projection	displacement
undoing	compensation
identification	denial

In Section II, we discuss growth and development theories as presented by a number of theorists. Freud in particular believed that most humans use **defense mechanisms** to some extent. He considered these to be ways of coping with anger or frustration or dealing with possible failure and loss of self-respect. Today, some psychologists believe that the use of defense mechanisms may block or stifle psychological growth. Others believe they are necessary for survival and they indeed protect us from what we cannot yet face.

The term *defense mechanisms* has been defined as behavior that is used to protect the ego from guilt, anxiety, or loss of esteem. Using defense mechanisms is a process that the unconscious uses to combat and fight anxiety. It is the body's way of seeking relief or guarding itself from uncomfortable feelings.

An individual wishing to block an emotionally painful experience may subconsciously or consciously use a defense mechanism. This enables the individual to put a problem on hold until sufficient time has elapsed to work through the situation and arrive at a solution, or come to terms of acceptance.

The use of defense mechanisms may be healthy or unhealthy. It may be considered an unhealthy approach if the problem is never resolved. Behavior resulting from the use of defense mechanisms may be inappropriate in later developmental stages. An example might be the child who throws a temper tantrum in an effort to get the parents' attention. Then, during early school years, this same child becomes the class clown to seek attention from those in authority.

The use of defense mechanisms is difficult to analyze since it is the motive behind the behavior that characterizes the various mechanisms and gives them their individuality. Some mechanisms may be used to provide time to adjust and accept a problem, while others may be used to cope or survive a situation. Some commonly used defense mechanisms are described in the following paragraphs.

Regression

Regression is an attempt to go back to an earlier stage of development to escape fear, anxiety, or conflict. This defense mechanism may be used by toddlers who have been toilet-trained for a year or two. When a new baby arrives in the household, toddlers may become anxious or feel displaced and regress to soiling themselves again. The foreign-born geriatric client who experiences hospitalization and is very anxious and fearful may regress to speaking in the native language. Regression is an attempt to withdraw from a circumstance that is unpleasant in some way by retreating to an earlier, more secure stage of life.

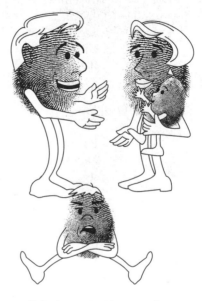

"I don't want to take a nap."

Repression

Repression is a method of defending by forgetting or experiencing temporary amnesia. It is the mind's way of protecting itself until it can cope with the overwhelming circumstance at the present time. The diabetic client who is to make an appointment for reevaluation in six months may "forget" to follow through. Another example of repression would be the child who fails a test and "forgets" to tell the parents. The consequences of not complying with the diabetic diet or the fear of how the parents may respond to the failing grade are overwhelming. By temporarily "forgetting" this emotionally painful consequence, the individual can go on with day-to-day activities. Clients with post-traumatic stress syndrome may use repression to deal with things too painful to face.

Sublimination

Sublimination involves the redirecting of a socially unacceptable impulse into a socially desirable behavior. An example would be the artist who expresses sexual impulses in sculpture or paintings. The physician may suggest that a childless couple whose choice is not to adopt children become involved in a hobby of breeding dogs or cats. Unmarried individuals wishing for children may substitute this desire by becoming day-care center workers.

Projection

Projection is attributing one's own thoughts or impulses to another individual as if they had originated in the other person. This is a form of defending oneself against feelings or urges that one does not want to admit are present. Usually negative or unacceptable feelings or urges are projected. A client may say "You're not really very helpful or caring" when in fact, it is the client who is not caring or sensitive to others. Projection may often be exhibited by mentally ill clients.

Displacement

Displacement is shifting the emotional element of a situation from a threatening object to a nonthreatening one. An example might be the client who is very angry with the physician for not explaining a procedure completely. When the client leaves the office, the door is slammed really hard, when in reality, the physician is being slammed.

Undoing

Undoing is to cancel out a behavior or try to make amends. In undoing, the individual is trying to make up for an inappropriate behavior and the guilty feelings that accompany the act. An abusive person often showers the abused with gifts after the abusive event hoping to "undo" the unacceptable behavior.

Compensation

Compensation is consciously or unconsciously overemphasizing a characteristic to compensate for a real or imagined deficiency. Compensation involves substituting a strength for a weakness and may be viewed as a healthy defense mechanism. For example, the young boy whose physical stature may keep him from being a football star may compensate by achieving an academic award.

Identification

Identification is unconsciously mimicking another's traits and behaviors in order to cope with feelings of inferiority or low self-image. This defense mechanism is often seen in adolescent clients as they begin to identify with groups and peers. They feel they must conform to the current trends and styles. Being different is considered unacceptable and may lead to being ignored or excluded from a particular group.

Denial

Denial is the unconscious refusal to acknowledge painful realities, feelings, or experiences. It offers a temporary escape from the unpleasant event. Often persons experiencing a heart attack will display denial. They describe the discomfort or pain as "just indigestion." Or when a laboratory report comes back positive and the client is told, they may express denial by saying "There must be a mistake!" Denial and repression are very similar and are considered the same by some authorities.

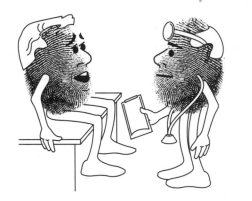

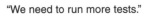

"There must be some mistake!"   "We need to run more tests."

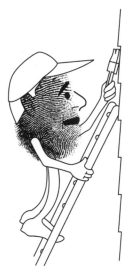

"I don't have time to think
about tests now."

Rationalization

Rationalization is the mind's way of justifying behavior by offering an explanation other than a truthful response. It is often used to save face or avoid embarrassment. There is usually some grain of truth tied to the explanation. The client told by the physical therapist to exercise the neck several times a day for five minutes may respond with an excuse such as "I couldn't do the exercises that often because I had to go to work." Actually, the client could have completed the exercises while seated at a desk. It was true that the client did have to continue to earn a living; however, this alone would not prevent following suggested treatment protocol.

———

Relying on defense mechanisms is automatic in adulthood, therefore, the mechanisms are often difficult to recognize. Taking a critical look at oneself, however, and trying to determine defenses used can lead to more effective ways of coping in the future.

Exercise 1

Review the list of defense mechanisms. Identify the one you use most often. List three instances when you used it in the last two weeks and what were the results.

Resources

1. Insel, Paul M. "Changing Your Self-Concept," *Healthline*, December, 1995, Vol. 14 Issue 12.

2. Kalman, Natalie, and Claire G. Waughfield. *Mental Health Concepts*, 4th ed. (Albany, NY: Delmar Publishers, 1998).

3. Navarra, Tova, Myron A. Lipowitz, and John G. Navarra. *Therapeutic Communication.* Thorofare, NJ: Slack, Inc. 1990.

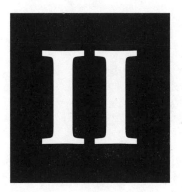

Learning Theories of Growth and Development

Chapter 5

Cognitive Development Learning Theory

Procedural Goal

To assist the student in identifying and understanding the importance of cognitive development and to relate Piaget's theory to therapeutic communications.

Learning Objectives

Upon completion of this unit, when given a written examination, the student will respond with a minimum of _____% accuracy within the defined class period for the exam.

- Describe Jean Piaget's theory of cognitive development.
- List Piaget's four stages of cognitive development.
- Identify examples of development that occur in each of the four stages of cognitive development.
- Discuss examples of the use of Piaget's theory of cognitive development in therapeutic communication.

Introduction

To be effective in therapeutic communications, one must have at least a basic understanding of human growth and development and psychology. The health professional should have a sound background and understanding of biological human growth and development and must, of necessity, consider these principles when communicating with others.

To communicate therapeutically, helping professionals must consider a person's lifetime experiences, conditioning, predisposition and inherited characteristics, life cycle and span, relationship to others, learning abilities and vocation, and cultural background.

Many prominent theories of human growth and development and psychology will be introduced in this chapter. Others have not been included. Of all the theories known, no *one* theory is generally accepted. Perhaps this is because, as Carl Rogers the psychotherapist believes, we are still in process. We are still learning and developing more viable and creative ways to live and work.

The goal of any health professional must be to enable individuals to get in touch with themselves to encourage them to discover a full and functioning life with meaning and purpose. Therefore, the more the health care professional knows and understands about human growth and development, the better prepared he/she will be to offer therapeutic communication.

Jean Piaget (1896–1980)

Jean Piaget (1896–1980) renowned Swiss psychologist, wrote volumes on his cognitive development theory and origins of knowledge in the child. Jean Piaget's theory of cognitive development states that motor activity involving concrete objects results in the development of mental functioning. For example, as an infant discovers his hand holding a rattle, he begins to recognize a sound that occurs every time he moves his hand with the rattle in it. Therefore, reflex activity drops out as repetition produces a result that the infant observes; his activity begins to take on purpose. Eventually, the infant identifies the shaking rattle as a producer of sound. Later, he will realize that he is able to create the sound.[1] Piaget felt that cognitive development came from the child's interaction with the environment. **Cognitive** refers to the ability to think and reason logically and to understand abstract ideas. Piaget states that as cognitive development progresses, children gain insights, learn to solve problems, and are able to understand abstract concepts. Some believe that Piaget's theory is as important to cognitive development as Sigmund Freud's theory is to psychiatry.

Piaget identified four stages or periods in which children progress in their learning.[2]

1. Sensorimotor activities: birth to two years of age
2. Preoperational thought: two to six years of age
3. Concrete operational thought: seven to eleven years of age
4. Formal operational thought: age 12 through adulthood

Sensorimotor Period (birth to about age 2)

As you might expect from the title of this period, a child's sensory and motor development are identified. According to Piaget, children in the sensorimotor stage only know the world through their senses and motor skills: in other words, their understanding of objects is limited to what their senses convey to them and what their motor skill development will permit them to perform. Because so much cognitive activity takes place during this period, Piaget divided the period into six separate stages.

- Stage 1 (birth to one month)—Sucking, an innate reflex activity, is paramount. The child does not differentiate between self and other objects.
- Stage 2 (one to four months)—The child begins to make distinctions, repeats simple actions, shows curiosity, and begins hand-to-mouth coordination.
- Stage 3 (four to eight months)—The child experiences increased manipulation and control of objects, repeats rewarding activities and develops eye-to-hand coordination.
- Stage 4 (eight to twelve months)—In the period just prior to the first birthday, the child imitates and anticipates events more actively and shows a growing sense of organization of things.

- Stage 5 (twelve to eighteen months)—This child explores and experiments more and discovers new ways to get what he/she wants.
- Stage 6 (eighteen to twenty-four months)—Begins to imagine things and speak words.

Preoperational Period (age 2 to about 6)

Following the sensorimotor period is the stage for preoperational thought, in which Piaget theorized that children are unable to understand logical concepts such as conversation, reversibility, or classification. At this age children begin to think symbolically, which is demonstrated through language formation, thinking of past and future events, and the ability to pretend and fantasize. This stage is divided into a **preconceptual** stage (two to four years) and an intuitive stage (four to six years). The years are approximations only. The child's thinking in this stage is egocentric or self-centered and the child believes everyone sees the world as the child sees it. Words are important and begin to stand for objects.

- The child focuses attention on only one aspect of a situation; cannot recognize two dimensions at the same time.
- Does not fully understand quantity, weight, length, volume.
- Cannot follow or fully understand reality as it changes.
- Thought is irreversible; cannot understand how something may change and then return to its original condition.

Period of Concrete Operations (7 to 11 years)

Children learn to perceive differences in sizes and volumes and are capable of reason. Yet they are not logical or adult in their thinking. Characteristics of this period include the following. The child:

- Is able to classify objects by category
- Becomes able to focus attention on more than one situation at a time
- Is able to distinguish length, quantity, and weight

- Begins to grasp changes in situations and to consider another's point of view
- Is able to understand that some things can be reversed

Period of Formal Operations (age 12 through adulthood)

This is the stage of adolescence and is characterized by hypothetical, logical, and abstract thought processes.

- Children in this stage recognize enough about the world to grasp abstract concepts. Most can arrive at several possible solutions when given a problem.
- Adolescents can conceive of ideas and concepts outside of their own experiences.
- A more mature notion of time develops and long-term goals can be set.
- A child is more fully able to understand symbols, such as those seen in political cartoons and algebra.
- Children tend to be idealistic; challenge adult decisions and authority figures.

Although some authorities will disagree with portions of Piaget's theories, his work has been very influential. According to Piaget's theory of cognitive development, each individual needs to make sense of new experiences by relating them with existing understanding. Therefore, every child progresses through each stage of development in the same sequence, however, the timetable may vary from one child to the next. Cognitive development is a continuing process as more of life is experienced. We should also remember that family, culture, personality, and socialization of the sexes may influence individual differences in cognitive development. Recognizing Piaget's developmental periods enables health professionals to communicate on a level to match a child's development and understanding. Sharing this information with parents who may be struggling to understand their child can also be beneficial.

The exercises at the end of this chapter will help you further understand Piaget's theory.

Exercise 1

If you have brothers or sisters or can observe children whose ages are identified in Piaget's period of growth and development, write a brief paper identifying at least five descriptions of activities performed by these children in those periods. Did you observe any children who were performing tasks prior to the age Piaget suggests? Later than suggested? What does this exercise tell you about how you can best communicate with each age group?

Exercise 2

Select two children from a family, day care, or preschool setting. One should be in the age group 4 to 7 years; the other should be between 7 and 11 years. Perform the following exercises.

Understanding of Length*

1. Get two sticks, pieces of yarn, or straws of the same length. Alone with each child, align your sticks, yarn, or straws in front of the child and ask if the items are equal in length. Observe the response. Now move one of your objects a little to the right of the other and ask the child if they are the same length. Observe the response.

*

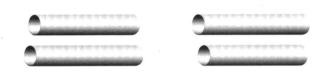

Understanding of Number**

2. Using ten pennies, align five pennies in two rows. Again alone with each child, ask if there is the same number of pennies in each row. Observe the response. Now move one row of pennies further apart and ask if there are the same number of pennies. Observe the response.

**

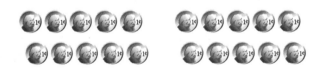

Understanding of Liquid Mass***

3. Fill two clear small round glasses of the exact size with the same amount of milk. Ask each child alone if the liquid in each glass is the same amount. Observe your response. Now pour the milk from one the glasses into a glass of a size taller and more slender in shape. Ask if the glasses now hold the same amount of milk. Observe your response.

***

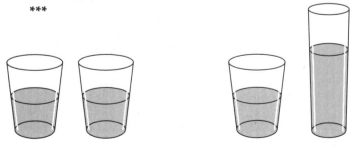

What have you learned from these experiments? Planning the experiments and deciding how to communicate with each child is part of the exercise. Were the children able to understand your instructions? Did they ask for explanations? Was your communication level appropriate for the ages?

What periods of cognitive development most correctly identify your children's reactions?

Endnotes

1. Barbara Schoen Johnson. *Psychiatric-Mental Health Nursing Adaptation and Growth,* 2nd ed. (Philadelphia: J.B. Lippincott Co., 1989), 49.

2. Kathleen Stassen Berger, and Ross A. Thompson. *The Developing Person through the Life Span.* (New York, NY: Worth Publishers, 1998), 40.

Resources

1. Berger, Kathleen Stassen, and Thompson, Ross A. *The Developing Person Through the Life Span.* New York, NY: Worth Publishers, 1998.

2. Frisch, Noreen Cavan, and Lawrence E. Frisch. *Psychiatric Mental Health Nursing.* Albany, New York: Delmar Publishers, 1998.

3. Johnson, Barbara Schoen. *Psychiatric-Mental Health Nursing Adaptation and Growth,* 4th ed. (Philadelphia: Lippincott-Raven, 1996).

Chapter 6

Psychoanalytic Development Learning Theories

Procedural Goal

To enhance the student's understanding of therapeutic approaches throughout the life span in terms of psychosocial theories of human growth and development.

Learning Objectives

Upon completion of this unit, when given a written examination, the student will respond to the following with a minimum of ____% accuracy within the defined class period for the exam.

- Describe Sigmund Freud's psychosocial forces—the id, the ego, and the superego.
- Define erogenous zones and name them.
- List the five psychosexual developmental stages as presented by Freud.
- Differentiate Erikson's eight stages of psychosocial development, being able to associate various tasks and therapeutic approaches that accompany each stage.

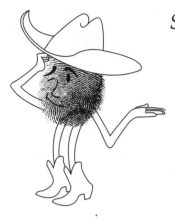

"Id, Ego, Superego?"

Sigmund Freud (1856–1939)

Sigmund Freud, a Viennese physician, developed the pscho-analytic theory which stresses irrational and unconscious forces that are hidden from our awareness and underlie human behavior. His theory focuses on pychosexual development and emphasizes that each stage must be conquered before progressing to the next stage. Freud theorized that each individual's behavior consists of three major systems or forces. These he called the **id**, the **ego**, and the **superego**. In the mentally healthy person these three forces work together cooperatively and enable the individual to realize fulfillment of basic needs and desires. When the three systems are at odds with one another, persons are said to be maladjusted.

The Id

Freud identified the id as a person's basic animal nature. It is primarily unconscious and is amoral. It is not governed by laws of reason or logic, and possesses no values or ethics. The id's primary function is to decrease pain and increase pleasure—also known as the **pleasure principle**.

In its earliest form, the id is a reflex response. For example, when a bright light falls on the retina of the eye, the eyelid closes and light is prevented from reaching the retina. The excitations produced in the nervous system by the light can then quiet down to maintain homeostasis.

An example of an internal reflex occurs when a valve in the bladder opens as the pressure on it reaches a certain intensity. The excitation or tension produced by the pressure ends as the contents of the bladder are emptied.

The id retains its infantile character throughout life. It cannot tolerate tension. It wants immediate gratification. It is demanding, impulsive, irrational, selfish, and pleasure-loving. It is the spoiled child personality. The pursuit of pleasure and the avoidance of pain are the only functions that count. It does not think, it only wishes or acts.

The Ego

The ego is the psychological force that is in touch with reality and mediates between the id and the superego. It deals with the outside world in a conscious fashion. The ego is governed by the **reality principle**, reality meaning that which exists. The goal of the reality principle is to postpone the discharge of energy until the actual object that will satisfy the need has been discovered or produced. For instance, we must learn to delay gratification (for example, eating when we are hungry, sleeping when we are tired, and so on) until the timing or the situation is appropriate for fulfillment of our needs.

This delay of action means that the ego has to be able to tolerate tension until it can be discharged in an appropriate form of behavior. The institution of the reality principle does not mean that the pleasure principle is forsaken. It is only temporarily suspended. Eventually, the reality principle leads to pleasure, although a person may have to endure some discomfort while looking for reality.

The ego's lines of development are laid down by heredity and guided by natural growth processes. This means that every person has inborn potential for thinking and reasoning that come through experience, training, and education.

The Superego

The superego is the moral branch of the personality. It represents the ideal rather than the real. It strives for perfection rather than reality or pleasure. The superego is the person's moral code. It develops out of the ego as a consequence of the child's assimilation of his/her parents' or primary caregivers' standards regarding what is good and virtuous and what is bad and sinful.

The superego is made up two groups, the **ego-ideal** and the **conscience**. The ego-ideal corresponds to the child's conceptions of what his/her parents or primary caregivers consider to be morally good. The standards of virtue are conveyed to children by rewards given for conduct in line with those standards. If they are consistently rewarded for being neat and tidy, then neatness is apt to become one of their ideals.

Conscience, on the other hand, corresponds to the child's conceptions of what his/her parents or primary caregivers feel is morally bad as established through experiences with punishment. If children have been frequently punished for getting dirty, then dirtiness is considered to be something bad.

Freud's Erogenous Zones

Some regions of the body are more likely to experience tensions that can be relieved by some action upon the region, such as sucking or stroking. These areas are referred to as **erogenous zones**. Manipulation of an erogenous zone is satisfying because it affords relief from irritation (such as scratching relieves an itching sensation) and because it induces a pleasurable sensual feeling.

The principal erogenous zones are the mouth, the anus, and the genital organs. Each of the principal zones is associated with the satisfaction of a vital need: the mouth with eating, the anus with elimination, and the sex organs with reproduction, Table 6-1.

Freud maintained that the erogenous zones are of great importance for the development of personality since they are the first sources of tension the infant has to contend with, and they yield the first important experiences of pleasure.

Psychosexual Stages

Freud proposed a theory of childhood sexuality in which psychosexual stages were identified. Each stage is characterized by the focus on a specific erogenous zone and the pleasure derived from that particular body part.

Table 6-1 Freud's Stages of Psychosexual Development

Stage	Age Range	Erogenous Zone	Sexual Activity
Oral	birth to one year	mouth, lips, tongue	sucking, swallowing, chewing, biting
Anal	one to three years	anus, buttocks	expulsion and retention of waste products
Phallic (Oedipus)	three to six years	genitals	masturbation
Latent	seven to eleven years	genitals	masturbation
Genital (Oedipus)	twelve+ years	genitals	masturbation, sexual intercourse, feeling for others

Oral Stage (birth to one year)

During the oral stage, Freud believed the infant derived greatest sensual satisfaction through the mouth. Oral activities — such as nursing from the mother's breast or the nipple of a bottle, sucking the thumb, or biting object placed in the infant's mouth—provide maximal pleasure and gratification.

At this stage of development, the infant is basically controlled by biological impulses and completely dependent upon others for basic needs. According to Freud, if these drives are not sufficiently satisfied in infancy, certain oral traits—such as overeating, excessive smoking or talking, or "having a biting tongue"—may be observed in the adult.

Anal Stage (one to three years)

At the other end of the alimentary canal is the anus, through which the solid waste products of digestion are eliminated from the body. Tensions arise in this region as a result of accumulation of fecal material. This material exerts pressure upon the walls of the colon. When the pressure upon the anal sphincters reaches a certain level, they open and the waste products are expelled by the act of defecation.

Expulsion brings relief to the person as the source of tension is removed. As a consequence of experiencing pleasurable tension-reduction from elimination, this mode of action may be employed to get rid of tensions that arise in other parts of the body. Expulsive elimination is the prototype for emotional outbursts, temper tantrums, rages, and other primitive discharge reactions.

During the second year of life or earlier, the involuntary expulsion reflexes are brought under voluntary control with toilet training. This time period can be viewed as a power struggle between child and parent. Retention (holding back the feces) may occur, and is viewed as a defense against the loss of something that is considered valuable. The gentle pressure on the internal walls of the rectum by the fecal material is also sensual satisfying. Defecation terminates this pleasure and leaves a feeling of depletion and emptiness. If a person fixates on this form of erotic pleasure it may develop into a generalized interest in collecting, possessing, and retaining objects.

Individuals naturally resist having a pleasurable activity interfered with and regulated. If the interference is very strict and punitive, children may retaliate intentionally by soiling themselves. As these children grow older, they may get even with frustrating authority figures by being messy, irresponsible, disorderly, wasteful, and extravagant. Strict toilet-training procedures may also bring about a reaction against uncontrolled expulsiveness in the form of meticulous neatness, fastidiousness, compulsive orderliness, frugality, disgust, fear of dirt, or strict budgeting of time and money.

Phallic/Oedipus Stage (three to six years)

The period of growth during which children are preoccupied with their genitals is called the **phallic** or **Oedipus** stage. During this stage, children identify with and desire sensual satisfaction from the parent of the opposite sex and view the parent of the same sex as a rival. This is the time when many young children discover the pleasures of masturbation.

Latent Stage (seven to eleven years)

The child identifies with the parent of the same sex in this stage and learns to assume the appropriate social role. During this stage, sexual drives are relatively quiet since they have come under the censorship of the conscience.

Genital Stage (twelve+ years)

Adolescents derive their most pleasurable experiences through the genital organs. An attraction to members of the opposite sex occurs. It is a period of socialization, group activities, marriage, establishing a home and raising a family, development of a serious interest in vocational advancement, and other adult responsibilities. It is the longest stage of the four, lasting from the late teens until old age.

————

The crux of Freud's theory is that each individual must successfully resolve the needs and conflicts of each stage in order to pass successfully into the succeeding stage. The problem, however, according to Freud, is that many people do not reach the fulfillment of the genital stage. If they have not successfully mastered the challenges of the earlier stages, they are prey to a variety of emotional symptoms and personality problems.

Even though many authorities today do not accept Freud's ideas word for word, his concepts have been immensely influential. They are the foundation of the work of many present-day psychoanalytic practitioners and theorists.

Erik Erikson (1902–1994)

Erikson spent his childhood in Germany, his adolescence wandering through Italy, his young adulthood in Austria working with Freud, and his later life in the United States. In America, he studied a wide variety of subjects, including students at Harvard, soldiers who suffered emotional breakdowns during World War II, civil rights workers in the South, disturbed and normal children at play, and Native American tribes. Until his death in 1994, he continued to write and lecture on psychosocial development.[1] Erikson is the foremost proponent of **ego psychology**, the psychoanalytic study of the self. His stress is not on emotional illness but on the individual's opportunities to triumph over the psychological hazards of daily life.

Like Freud, Erikson teaches that psychological development is a continuous process, each phase or stage a part of a continuum. Each developmental stage presents a problem or crisis that the individual must face and master. These **psychosocial crises** are conflicts between a person and society or social institutions. They are the motivating forces behind the individual's behavior. Resolution of each life crisis enhances a person's ability to meet the next crisis and is characterized by hypothetical, logical, and abstract thought processes.

The eight psychosocial crises of Erikson are described in Table 6–2.

Trust Versus Mistrust (Infancy)

When infants' needs are met in a consistent and affectionate manner, they are satisfied that their world is a safe place. Trust is built. When those basic needs are not recognized and met, mistrust develops.

Tasks involved during this stage include the parent and infant adjusting to each other, and the infant learning to take solid foods, to walk, and to talk.

Table 6-2 Erikson's Psychosocial Crises

Pyschosocial Crisis	Age Range	Positive Outcome
Trust versus Mistrust	Infancy Birth to eighteen months	Physical comfort and security
Autonomy versus Shame and Doubt	Toddlers eighteen months to three years	Ability to hold on (dependency) and to let go (autonomy)
Initiative versus Guilt	Preschool three to six years	Initiative to master new tasks
Industry versus Inferiority	School Years six to eleven years	Productivity and mastery of skills
Identity versus Role Confusion	Adolescence eleven to eighteen years	Ability to be oneself
Intimacy versus Isolation	Early Adulthood eighteen to thirty-five years	Capacity for affiliation and love
Generativity versus Stagnation	Middle Adulthood thirty-five to sixty-five years	Concern for the succeeding generation
Integrity versus Despair	Late Adulthood sixty-five+ years	Sense of fulfillment with one's life

Autonomy Versus Shame and Doubt (Toddlers)

During this stage, children either develop a sense of pride in their independence and new accomplishments or they develop feelings of shame and doubt concerning their ability to deal with other people and the world.

Tasks accomplished during this stage include children seeking independence in their actions, learning to control elimination, learning to communicate through language, and learning to differentiate between right and wrong.

Initiative Versus Guilt (Preschool)

In this stage, children learn to initiate activities. It is the response they receive to these activities that determines whether their sense of initiative will remain intact or whether they will feel a sense of guilt for their actions.

Tasks learned are establishing relations with peers, beginning to form concepts based on reality, refining motor control, and learning a social role based on gender identification.

Industry Versus Inferiority (School Years)

During this stage, children divide their time between home and school. A negative response received at home to their new sense of industry can be neutralized by a positive response at school, or vice versa. If the child encounters consistent failure or discouragement, however, he/she will experience feelings of inferiority.

Tasks accomplished during this phase include learning autonomy, refining coordination, learning cooperation and self-control, developing social skills, learning to view the world objectively, and forming values of their own.

Identity Versus Role Confusion (Adolescence)

During this stage, the adolescent ideally develops a positive and stable sense of identity or self-image in relation to the past and future. Lacking this, children will experience a sense of confusion with regard to their social role.

Tasks learned include the adolescent accepting a changing physique, seeking and achieving independence from adults, forming close peer relations, defining social roles, and beginning to reason logically.

Intimacy Versus Isolation (Early Adulthood)

During this stage, individuals establish close relationships with others. If individuals are not close to anyone, they will experience feelings of isolation.

Tasks include selecting a career path, choosing a partner, raising children, and assuming social responsibilities.

Generativity Versus Stagnation (Middle Adulthood)

Generativity means being concerned with the future of society and the world in general. Middle-aged adults have raised their family, contribute to the community and their place of employment, are involved in various levels of government, and enjoy many meaningful activities. Individuals lacking these fulfillments become overly concerned with themselves and stagnate.

Tasks accomplished during this stage include adjusting to physical and physiological changes, accepting the needs of their children and of their aging parents, and attaining career and social goals.

Integrity Versus Despair (Late Adulthood)

During this stage, most adults take stock of their lives and accomplishments. If they are content with what they have done, they experience what is called **ego integrity**, a sense of wholeness. Adults who are dissatisfied with their lives, who wish they could do it over again yet know that it is impossible, succumb to despair.

Tasks accomplished include the individual accepting the aging process, adjusting to retirement, and adjusting to the death of partner and/or friends.

The following, Table 6-3, may be helpful in further understanding growth and development according to Eric Erikson's psychosocial development and its relationship in the medical office.

Table 6-3 Psychosocial Development According to Eric Erikson

Age	Developmental Stage	Therapeutic Approach
	Trust versus Mistrust	
Birth to four weeks	*Motor Development:* Visual fixation (stares at windows and ceiling), eyes follow bright moving objects, head sags when unsupported, makes crawling movements when prone. *Physical Growth:* Gains 5 to 7 ounces weekly and grows one inch monthly (for 6 months). *Vocalization:* Cries when hungry or uncomfortable making throaty sounds. Tries to communicate pain or discomfort.	The infant is dependent on others. It is important to provide time for parents to talk about their feelings and ask questions. Health professional should smile and use a pleasant, calm voice. Encourage parents to verbalize feelings and concerns and respond to each inquiry.
Two months	*Motor Development:* Eyes are better controlled, can turn body from side to back, can hold head erect, in midposition. *Physical:* Growth pattern continues; posterior fontanel closed. *Vocalization:* Knows crying will get attention; crying becomes differentiated—such as for hunger, pain, attention. *Socialization:* Begins to respond to attention by expressing a "social smile" in response to others.	Mobiles over the examination table create a pleasing atmosphere for the infant. Respond to the "social smile." Remember, infants of this age can roll off the table or counter, so never leave them unattended or take your eyes or hands off them.

Table 6-3 (Continued)

Age	Developmental Stage	Therapeutic Approach
Three months	*Motor Development:* When prone will rest on forearms and keep head midline; discovers and stares at hands; plays with hands and fingers; able to place hand or object in mouth at will. *Vocalization:* Babbles and coos, laughs aloud; shows pleasure in making sounds; makes initial vowel sounds. *Socialization:* Recognizes parent or primary caregiver.	Use caution in regard to what is within reach of infants as they are much more active at this stage. The infant recognizes familiar faces or voices, so include parent and/or primary caregiver in procedures where appropriate.
Four months	*Motor Development:* Holds head up; can turn body from back to side; recognizes familiar objects, sits with adequate support. *Physical:* Drools (does not know how to swallow saliva); deciduous teeth appear. *Vocalization:* Vocalizes socially (coos when talked to)—very talkative. *Socialization:* Enjoys having people close by; initiates social play by smiling.	Use caution in regard to what is within reach or on the floor—everything goes into the mouth. Continue to formulate a positive experience with the child.
Six months	*Motor Development:* Reaches for objects, grasps objects with whole hand, can hold two objects—one in either hand; can pull self to sitting position; turns over stomach to back; bangs objects in hand; hitches for locomotion. *Physical:* Doubles birth weight, continues to gain 3 to 5 ounces weekly and grows one-half inch monthly. *Vocalization:* Vocalizes displeasure, vocalizes several distinguishable syllables; cries easily. *Socialization:* Begins to recognize strangers.	Safety measures must be exercised. Smile when talking to children of this age. Provide a warm and friendly atmosphere.
Eight months	*Motor Development:* Bounces and bears some weight when held in standing position; discovers feet; hand-eye coordination is perfected; sits alone; displays exploratory behaviors with food. *Vocalization:* Makes polysyllabic vowel sounds, imitates speech sounds. *Socialization:* Shows fear of strangers and affection for family.	The child is developing a memory and has some ability to think. Wearing colored uniform tops or jackets or buttons for interest may be helpful. Smile often and "talk" to the child.

(continued)

Table 6-3 (Continued)

Age	Developmental Stage	Therapeutic Approach
Ten months	*Motor Development:* Crawls and creeps; raises self to sitting position; sits alone; preference for use of one hand; manipulates objects; can hold bottle and feed self cookie; can control lips around cup. *Vocalization:* Says one or two words; is able to initiate expression and gestures. *Socialization:* Pays attention to his/her name; plays simple games (bye-bye, pat-a-cake); responds to adult anger (tone of voice).	Involve child in simple games; be aware of the tone of voice used; when child is eating, use care to prevent choking.
Twelve months	*Motor Development:* Stands alone for a moment; walks with help; can sit from standing position without help; can pick up food and transfer to mouth; cooperates in dressing. *Physical:* Triples birth weight; doubles birth length. *Vocalization:* Uses expressive jargon, recognizes meaning of "no-no." *Socialization:* Still egocentric; shows emotions (jealousy, affection, anxiety and anger); responds to music.	Use praise and rewards to reinforce positive behavior. May play music in exam room. Allow the child to help dress after a procedure.
Twelve to fifteen months	*Motor Development:* Walks alone; can release objects at will; tells parent or primary caregiver "I do it"; gets into things; has one directional thinking—mine, no-no. *Physical:* **Babinski** and **Landau** reflexes disappear. *Vocalization:* Points to indicate wants. *Socialization:* Shares emotions; enjoys being center of attention.	The key element is *safety.* Use large blocks, stuffed toys that are washable, cloth books in the reception area and examination room. Do not keep children and parents waiting long; excessive wait encourages anxiety.

Table 6-3 (Continued)

Age	Developmental Stage	Therapeutic Approach
	Autonomy versus Shame and Doubt	
Toddler (Eighteen to twenty-four months)	*Motor Development:* Walks up and down stairs; opens doors; turns knobs; uses spoon without spilling; helps undress self; can jump. *Vocalization:* Knows 200 to 300 words, begins to use short sentences. *Socialization:* Obeys simple commands; uses word "mine" constantly; enjoys parallel play (health professional plays with a puppet while the child plays with a puppet also).	Use simple commands, such as "roll over," and "give me the book." Reward acceptable behavior with hugs and stamps on the hand.
Two to three years	*Motor Development:* Feeds self well; can undress self; walks backwards; begins to use scissors. *Physical:* Has full set of 20 deciduous teeth. *Vocalization:* Knows 900 words. *Socialization:* Negativism grows out of child's sense of developing independence. Rituals are important.	Develop a consistent routine for office visits. Provide rewards for positive behavior. Talk to the child directly as much as possible.
	Initiative versus Guilt	
Preschool (Three to six years)	*Motor Development:* Dresses self (buttons and ties shoelaces); climbs and jumps well. *Physical:* Growth is relatively slow (gains less than 5 pounds per year and grows 2 to 2 $^1/_2$ inches per year). *Socialization:* Health professionals may find it helpful to have the child alone in the examination room. Talks to imaginary friends; can be given simple explanation as to cause and effect; still needs security of parent's presence. Initial need to be accepted by others outside the family; strong motivation to measure up.	Give simple explanations and short, simple commands. This age group responds well to drawings and play. May give a pretend injection to doll and explain, "This will hurt for a minute. It will help you feel better so you can play happily."

(continued)

Table 6-3 (Continued)

Age	Developmental Stage	Therapeutic Approach
	Industry versus Inferiority	
Adolescence (Six to eleven years)	*Motor Development:* Coordination is refined; begins to develop independence; likes to bathe self without assistance.	Provide encouragement and praise where appropriate. Encourage self-esteem. Explain procedures at the child's level. Provide choices where appropriate: "Should I see how tall you are first or how much you weigh?"
	Physical: Height increases proportionally to weight gain; begins to lose baby teeth; acquires first molars.	
	Socialization: Begins to take responsibility for own actions; begins to accept authority outside the home; uses the telephone; works for acceptance; has to be good at something or feels inferior; no interest in the opposite sex.	
	Identity versus Role Confusion	
Eleven to eighteen years	*Motor Development:* Awkward.	Peer importance is critical. Provide privacy and remember this group is very modest. They have a fear of losing their independence. They have a fear and concern regarding future changes in body image: Will this procedure or process impact future activity levels?
	Physical: Females—menstruation begins; axillary and pubic hair becomes coarser and darker; increased development of breasts. Males—grow pubic and facial hair; growth spurt, that is, height, shoulders broaden; voice changes; axillary hair develops; production of **spermatozoa, nocturnal emission** may occur. Both males and females—**sebaceous glands** on face, back, and chest become more active.	
	Socialization: Increased interest in the opposite sex; concerned with morality, ethics; peer group important; emancipation from family begins.	

"So doc, can I still play basketball?"

Table 6-3 (Continued)

Age	Developmental Stage	Therapeutic Approach
	Intimacy versus Isolation	
Early Adulthood (Eighteen to thirty-five years)	This group is interested in the development of a career, searching for a mate, and establishing a home and family. *Physical:* In general, experiencing good health and at their peak. Usually only routine examinations, or emergency care for an injury or illness is all that will be needed.	At this stage, individuals are self-confident and able to make rational decisions regarding their health care. Provide options and describe the benefits and expectations.
	Generativity versus Stagnation	
Middle (Thirty-five to sixty-five years)	This can be the most productive period as individuals are making and discovering new things. Usually established socioeconomically and do not have to struggle. Begin to think of charity; give back to their parents and community. *Physical:* Health maintenance is important during this stage. Routine examinations and procedures need to be evaluated regularly. A balanced diet and exercise program should be maintained. Attention should be given to stress levels and how to cope with stress in life experiences.	If these clients are not fulfilled, they will feel empty and dissatisfied. They either feel good about the past or they despair. Often they will brag of past accomplishments, reasserting worth. Listen to what they have to say. Provide health care choices when appropriate.
	Ego-Integrity versus Despair	
Adulthood (Sixty-five+ years)	These individuals are beginning to think of retirement or have retired; looking back on their lives and accomplishments. they may be afraid to die or may feel they have not lived life to its fullest. *Physical:* The body or mind or both may begin to fail. Body functions begin to decrease and/or malfunction.	Give these individuals a firm handshake and eye contact; address them by their full name and title; ask their opinion; allow them to make decisions regarding their health care if possible. Do not refer to them by using endearing terms such as "dear," "sweetie," or "honey."

"I just don't move as fast as I used to."

———

In physician offices today, we may not necessarily refer to these stages of growth and development as Erikson's. However, we certainly implement and incorporate the stages during client assessment and the helping interview sessions. An understanding of how the human body grows and develops is of great value in relating to clients and assisting their understanding and acceptance of the stages.

Exercise 1

Identify at least five experiences you have had with individuals you could identify as being in one of either Freud's or Erikson's stages of psychosocial development. What actions or evidence helped you make your decision? In a health care setting, how would you communicate therapeutically?

Endnotes

1. Kathleen Stassen Berger, and Ross A. Thompson. *The Developing Person through the Life Span* (New York, NY: Worth Publishers, 1998), 32.

Resources

1. Berger, Kathleen Stassen, and Ross A. Thompson. *The Developing Person through the Life Span.* New York, NY: Worth Publishers, 1998.

2. Erikson, Erik H., Joan M. Erikson, and Helen Q. Kivnick. *Vital Involvement in Old Age.* New York, NY: W. W. Norton and Co., 1994.

3. Frisch, Noreen Cavan, and Lawrence E. Frisch. *Psychiatric Mental Health Nursing.* Albany, New York: Delmar Publishers, 1998.

4. Johnson, Barbara Schoen. *Psychiatric-Mental Health Nursing.* Philadelphia: Lippincott-Raven, 1996.

Chapter 7

Moral Development Learning Theories

Procedural Goal

To assist the student in recognizing the moral development theories and to help the health care professional incorporate these theories into therapeutic communications.

Learning Performance Objectives

Upon completion of this unit, when given a written examination, the student will respond to the following with a minimum of _____% accuracy within the defined class period for the exam.

- Identify individuals in one's life most likely to influence moral development.
- Describe the six dimensions of moral development outlined by Jean Piaget.
- Describe the three stages of moral development outlined by Lawrence Kohlberg.
- Compare/contrast Paiget's and Kohlberg's outlines.
- Discuss appropriate methods health care professionals might use to encourage a healthy lifestyle as part of moral development.

Moral development is lifelong. When a toddler grabs a toy and says "mine" or when an elderly adult consciously signs a living will, moral behavior is exercised. The greatest growth in moral development occurs during adolescence. Between the ages of 10 to 20, individuals view moral issues more broadly.

Moral development is derived from a child's models. These include parents, caregivers, teachers, and peers. These models will, in part, determine the rules by which the child lives and develops a conscience. Once again, the work of Piaget is seen. He felt that cognitive development enabled a child to understand the relationship between models and their rules.

Piaget's Six Dimensions of Moral Development

Jean Piaget[1] identified six dimensions of moral development.

1. **Intentionality** — Is the intent related to the action? For example, is it more serious to accidentally break the lid of the cookie jar while stealing a cookie or to accidentally break a glass when drinking some milk? The younger child will not be able to a see a difference.

2. **Relativism** — A younger child thinks an action is totally right or totally wrong and that everyone has the same view. An older child will recognize that opinions may differ on what is right and what is wrong.

3. **Sanctions** — Children relate something bad not just by the punishment received. A young child thinks an action is bad if there is punishment related to it. The older child can determine the action without regard to **sanctions**. He/she can decide an act is bad because it violates a rule or is harmful.

4. **Reciprocity** — Young children do not understand "do unto others." If they do, it probably is in terms of "You hit me and I'll hit you back." It is not until a child is usually between the ages of 11 and 13 that the concept of putting oneself in the other's place begins to take hold.

5. **Restitution** — Punishment and reform is the focus here. A young child believes that the punishment is making up

for doing something wrong. As the child grows older, he/she favors more mild punishment or reform.

6. **Naturalistic** — Circumstances seen as beyond human control fall in this dimension. Younger children may think that falling off the bicycle and seriously scraping a knee is God's punishment for some earlier misdeed. Older children recognize the fallacy in this thinking.

It seems clear from Piaget's research that as children grow older they have a greater understanding of law and order and social convention.

Lawrence Kohlberg's Stages of Moral Development

Lawrence Kohlberg developed a theory that moral development is dependent upon the thinking and problem solving stimulated by the child. The theory claims that individuals acquire a sense of justice through a sequence of stages related to cognitive development. The stages closely parallel and are built on Piaget's theory and research.

Stages of Moral Development

I. *Preconventional Level*—avoid punishment and earn rewards

Stage 1. Punishment and reward are understood. To do good is to avoid punishment.

Stage 2. The idea of "you be good to me and I'll be good to you" develops.

II. *Conventional Level*

Stage 3. Moral behavior is what is accepted and approved by others. Approval becomes more important than reward.

Stage 4. Law and order and fixed rules are recognized, either by religion or social order or both.

III. *Postconventional, or Principled Level*

Stage 5. Actions are determined by individual rights or standards, such as the described laws and the United States Constitution. This is often considered to be the "social contract" stage.

Stage 6. Morality becomes individual principles that are logical, comprehensive, and consistent. Justice and equality of human rights, respect, and worthwhile life is recognized. Universal ethical principles are established.

The **preconventional level** is typical of children and delinquents. This level is described as **premoral** since most decisions are based on self-interest and materialism. The **conventional level** is the time when individuals believe social standards and laws are primary moral values. Kohlberg believes that the **postconventional** or **principled** level is when individuals follow moral reasoning that may supersede society's standards or their personal wishes.

Progression from one stage to another depends on a person's cognitive development and the opportunity to be exposed to different ideas and experiences. Standards change as society changes. As children grow older, however, discipline given in love seems to be more effective when encouraging moral development than is discipline that is aggressive and controlling.

Kohlberg's theory[2] more recently has been questioned by critics who identify the following:

- Kohlberg's original research used only boys, thus overlooking that females give greater consideration to the social content of moral choice. Females more easily look for a way to not have to judge right and wrong in absolute terms.

- Kohlberg's theories are built on universal "Western" values. In many non-Western cultures the good of the family and the community and their religious beliefs take precedence over all other considerations.

Even with the preceding criticism, however, it should be remembered that current research has also confirmed Kohlberg's overall scheme.

Role of Health Professionals

Health care professionals will not have a great influence on a child's moral development since so much of the development comes from those persons closest to the child. However, health care professionals will be called upon many times to care for a child when a discussion of a healthy lifestyle is appropriate. Positive reinforcement, praise, and verbal explanations should be used by health care professionals wishing to encourage a healthy lifestyle as part of normal development.

Consider, for example, the physician's office staff who distribute Mr. Yuk stickers for hazardous and poisonous materials and explain Mr. Yuk to children in the office. The physician's honest discussion with the adolescent about sex is another way to encourage a healthy lifestyle. Even adults need to be encouraged. An honest discussion about the effects of an unhealthy lifestyle continues throughout life.

Exercise 1

As you reflect upon moral development and the information in this chapter, you have probably been reminded of your own moral development. In a short report to be shared with your instructor, identify the individuals who were influential in your moral development. What is it that these people modeled for you? What other influences have been instrumental in moral development?

Try to identify **only five** beliefs you have about morality. You may have many more; however, try to determine which five would be the most important. Compare your list of five with others in class. Discuss what might cause these differences. Are the differences related to models? culture? religion?

Exercise 2

Consider one of Kohlberg's critic's identification that females view moral issues in a different manner then do males. Do you agree or disagree? Are you able to gives examples from your own experience to support your response?

Endnotes

1. Bernadine Chuck Fong. *The Child, Development through Adolescence.* (Menlo Park, CA: The Benjamin/Cummings Publishing Co., Inc. 1980), 395–396.

2. Kathleen Stossen Berger and Ross A. Thompson, *The Developing Person through the Life Span,* 4th ed. (New York, NY, Worth Publishers, 1998), 423.

Resources

1. Berger, Kathleen Strassen, and Ross A. Thompson. *The Developing Person through the Life Span,* 4th ed. (New York, NY, Worth Publishers, 1998).

2. Frisch, Noreen Cavan, and Lawrence E. Frisch. *Psychiatric Mental Health Nursing.* Albany, New York: Delmar Publishers, 1998.

Chapter 8

Behavioral and Humanistic Learning Theories

Procedural Goal

To assist the student to understand behavioral and humanistic theories of development and apply their importance to effective therapeutic communications.

Learning Objectives

Upon successful completion of this unit, when given a written examination, the student will respond to the following with a minimum of ____% accuracy within the defined class period for the exam.

- Name the two theorists who described conditional development.
- Describe Ivan Pavlov's famous dog experiment and discuss its relevance to therapeutic communications.
- Compare/contrast Pavlov's theory with Skinner's theory.
- Define positive reinforcement.
- Define negative reinforcement.
- Compare/contrast negative reinforcement with punishment.

- Name the humanist theorist who developed a hierarchy of needs.
- Identify each level of the hierarchy of needs and relate its relevance to therapeutic communications.

Learning theorists recognize that laws of behavior can be applied at any age. Learning theory explores the relationship between stimulus and response. If a hand is waved in your face, the response is automatic—you blink. If you panic each time your pass the corner where you were in a serious accident, the response is learned.

Life is a continuing process of learning. One part of this learning is knows as conditioning. Conditioning means that a particular stimulus or experience triggers a particular response.

Two theorists, Ivan Pavlov and B.F. Skinner, described how conditioning is critical to development. The two types of conditioning described are classical and operant. A brief discussion of these conditioned responses is helpful in further understanding of therapeutic communication.

Ivan Pavlov, Behaviorist

Ivan Pavlov[1], (1849–1936) Russian scientist, is well known for his identification of the earliest and simplest form of learning. He identified **classical conditioning** in his famous dog experiment which illustrates his theory. Pavlov knew that a dog salivated automatically as a reflex when there is food in its mouth. He presented food to the dog with the ringing of a loud bell. Eventually the bell alone caused the dog to salivate—the learned response. To further illustrate:

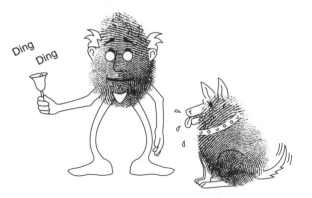

Example of Classical Conditioning

Unconditioned stimulus	=	**Unconditioned response**
—food		—salivation
Conditioning	=	Unconditioned response
—food and bell		—salivation
Conditioned stimulus	=	**Conditioned response**
—bell		—salivation

Health care professionals often experience this classical conditioning as seen by the small child who immediately begins to cry in fear when the assistant enters with a needle. The pain of the needle has been associated with the assistant so often that the child begins to cry just at the sight of the assistant. You may be able to relate similar responses. Some become quite anxious at the smell they associate with the dental office. Others are afraid when they see someone in a white uniform.

Health professionals remembering this conditioned response will consider methods to help alleviate this fear and anxiety. Employees in a pediatrics office might wear colors instead of white, even consider uniforms with children's figures on them. Making the experience as positive as possible will help. The physician might carry a toy or an object of distraction. He/she is advised to spend some time with a child in a nonthreatening manner. The physical setting should include objects that delight a child. Many find a built-in aquarium beneficial. Others use videos and children's tapes.

Even adults have conditioned responses and should be considered. A well-known cancer specialist, David Bressler, M.D., purchases juggling bags for his cancer clients. His primary goal is to make certain his clients have something other than the cancer, the pain, and the difficult treatment to associate with him. This physician teaches the client something new about juggling on each visit. They often juggle their bags together. Of course, added benefits are the laughter and the concentration on the juggling, which take the client's mind off the disease.

B.F. Skinner, Behaviorist

B.F. Skinner (1904–1990)[2] formulated the learning model knows as **operant conditioning**. Skinner and Pavlov agreed that classical conditioning explains some types of behavior. Skinner, however, believed that operant conditioning plays a much more important role.

The difference between classical conditioning and operant conditioning is that in operant conditioning, the response *precedes* the reward. For example, a rat pushes a lever and is rewarded with food. The food is pleasurable and useful, so the rat pushes the lever again. If the reward or consequences of pushing the lever is unpleasant, the rat will not repeat the behavior. Because a person's behavior is what brings the reward, this kind of conditioning may also be called **instrumental conditioning**.

Skinner believed that successful child rearing was accomplished through consistent rewarding of desirable behavior. If the behavior is followed by a pleasant reward or stimulus, the reinforcement is *positive*. If the behavior is followed by the removal of an unpleasant stimulus, the reinforcement is *negative*. Skinner believed that reinforcement was most effective if it is intermittent. Behavior would be rewarded most of the time, but not every time.

There are both *positive* and *negative reinforcements*. A positive reinforcement is something good or pleasant. A negative reinforcement is taking away the bad or unpleasant stimulus. Negative reinforcement is not to be confused with punishment. Punishment is an unpleasant event that makes behavior less likely to be repeated.

Remembering this theory is helpful in communicating. The little girl who is upset and crying because of the injection receives a badge of courage from the assistant for the injection site. As the child is being told how brave she was, and the badge is put on, she begins to feel better and a smile creeps across her face. This is an example of negative reinforcement.

The father who rewards his son with an ice-cream soda because he did such a good job raking the lawn, or the piano teacher who puts a gold star on the piece of music that was memorized are examples of positive reinforcement.

The reinforcement can be primary or secondary. A primary reinforcement is one that is basic and immediately satisfying, such as food. The reinforcement is secondary if the reward itself allows us to get something we want. An example of this is the allowance used as a reward that allows the child to go to the movies with a friend. It is also helpful to distinguish between negative reinforcement and punishment. In punishment, an unpleasant stimulus is applied to discourage behavior. Punishment may be necessary, but the child can also learn to avoid punishment without changing behavior. For example, a student who receives a failing grade on an exam may avoid the circumstances and skip class rather than fail again. Such behavior requires attention from anyone who has control over the circumstances. The teacher must award the grade earned by the student, but will try to create a positive and encouraging atmosphere for the student to study harder for the next test.

Social Learning Theory

Individuals also learn by observing the behavior of others. This observation is often called the social learning theory. A major part of social learning theory is modeling. In modeling, other people's behavior is observed and copied. This modeling occurs especially when we are uncertain of what is expected of us. When the behavior is modeled by someone we consider admirable or very important, we are likely to behave in the same way.

Children are especially sensitive to modeling. A young child wants to feed her doll just like mom feeds the new baby. With increasing age, we learn to be more discriminating in who and what behaviors we model.

In adulthood behavior is an outcome of reciprocal determination. This is when personal characteristics, the environment, personal expectations, self-perceptions, and goals determine behavior. For example, an extrovert responds differently than an introvert. An environment which is safe and encourages openness invokes that same behavior.

Abraham Maslow, Humanist

Abraham Maslow, born to Russian-Jewish immigrants in Brooklyn, New York, is considered the founder of humanistic psychology. However, he also considered himself to be a Freudian and a behaviorist. Maslow was not opposed to

Table 8-1 Maslow's Hierarchy of Needs

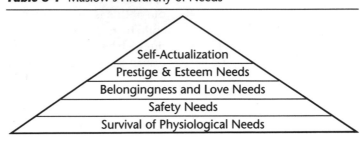

other theorists; he simply regarded his work as an extension of modern trends in psychology. He is well known for his **hierarchy** of needs, which is often used to illustrate motivating forces.

Maslow's[3] hierarchy of needs is illustrated in Table 8-1.

Maslow believed that if your basic *survival/physiological needs* were not met, it was not possible to consider needs for safety. Survival needs are identified as the need for food, water, and air to breathe—**homeostasis** for the body.

Safety needs are needs for security, stability, and protection. Everyone has the desire to be free from fear and anxiety. Safety needs also includes the need for structure, law and order, and limits.

The *belongingness and love needs* follow after safety needs are gratified. This level of need involves both giving and receiving affection. In this level, the true understanding of words used to describe our need for connectedness take on new meaning. Some of these words are roots, origins, peers, friends, family, neighborhood, territory, clan, class, and gang. We have a basic animal tendency to herd, flock, join, and belong.

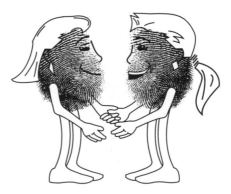

"You're my best friend."

The *esteem needs* come from a basic need for a stable, healthy self-respect for ourselves and others. There is the desire for achievement, strength, and confidence. Also, there is the need for recognition, prestige, reputation, status, even fame. Satisfaction of these needs leads to feelings of self-confidence and worth.

Once all the other needs have been met and realized, a person seeks **self-actualization**. Self-actualization has been identified as the peak time, a time when a person is doing truly what he or she is fitted for. It is an achievement of potential.

Individuals move back and forth from one need to another depending upon circumstances present at the time. It is helpful to recognize at what level of need a person is operating. If simple physiological needs are not being adequately met, it will be impossible for a physician to expect a client to purchase a medication that is necessary for proper treatment of an ailment.

Health care professionals alert to persons struggling from one level to another may be able to recommend or suggest community resources that can benefit clients whose life essentials or safety and security needs are not being met. Sometimes these individuals have serious problems and need outside assistance.

Counseling may be helpful if it appears that love and belonging needs are not met. This counseling might be individual or family in orientation. Helping individuals feel comfortable and giving them a sense of belonging to your health care facility is very therapeutic.

One last note on Maslow's theory. This theory clearly demonstrates that development continues throughout life. In this module, there appears to be much emphasis on the development of the child. Recognizing continuing development in the adult is equally important.

Conclusion

Many prominent theories of human growth and development and psychology have been introduced in this module. Others have not been included. Carl Rogers, the psychotherapist, believes we are still in process. We are still learning and developing more viable and creative ways to live and work.

The goal of any health professional must be to enable individuals to get in touch with themselves and encourage them to discover a full and functioning life with meaning and purpose.

Exercise 1

A client comes to the dental office in obvious pain and discomfort from a severely abscessed tooth. The client remarks, "I couldn't sleep, I can't eat, and I couldn't go to work today."

Which of Maslow's stages most accurately describes the client?

What action should the health professional take to assist this client?

Endnotes

1. Bernadine Chuck Fong, and Miriam Roher Resnick, *The Child, Development through Adolescence* (Menlo Park, CA: The Benjamin /Cummings Publishing Co., Inc., 1980), 262–264.

2. Kathleen Stassen Berger, and Ross A. Thompson, *The Developing Person through the Life Span,* 4th ed. New York, NY: Worth Publishers, 1998, 36.

Resources

1. Berger, Kathleen Stassen, and Ross A. Thompson. *The Developing Person through the Life Span,* 4th ed. (New York, NY: Worth Publishers, 1998).

2. Frisch, Noreen Cavan, and Lawrence E. Frisch. *Psychiatric Mental Health Nursing.* (Albany, New York: Delmar Publishers, 1998).

3. Maslow, Abraham H. *Motivation and Personality.* New York: Harper and Row, 1987.

4. Milliken, Mary Elizabeth. *Understanding Human Behavior: A Guide for Health Care Providers,* 6th ed. (Albany, NY: Delmar Publishers, 1998).

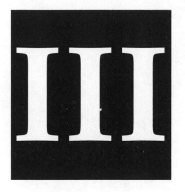

The Therapeutic Response

Chapter 9

The Therapeutic Response in Age Groups

Procedural Goal

To enhance the student's understanding of age-group differences in the use of therapeutic communications in the health care setting.

Learning Objectives

Upon completion of this unit, when given a written examination, the student will respond to the following with a minimum of _____% accuracy within the defined class period for the exam.

- Identify a minimum of five characteristics particular to children, to adolescents, to adults, and to elder adults.
- Describe at least four guidelines for therapeutic communication for each age group, giving an example of how each might be instituted.
- Discuss the concept that to be really therapeutic, health care professionals must genuinely like their work and the age groups they are treating.

Children

Katie is going to the doctor today. She is two-and-one-half years old. She is excited about going because they have such great toys for her. When she arrives with her Grandma, she goes straight for the toys. The wait is not long, and when the medical assistant is ready, she calls Katie by name. In the examination room, the physician talks directly to Katie, allows her to play with the stethoscope, and to listen to her heartbeat. Katie is not afraid and likes the physician.

———

Section II, "Learning Theories of Growth and Development," provided information about how children grow, develop, form their personalities, and become mature adults. Remembering these guidelines is beneficial for any health professional who wishes to be therapeutic.

Any person may have difficulty adjusting to being ill and to being under the care of a physician. Children may have an even more difficult time because they do not fully understand what is happening to them. Children cannot comprehend why the medicine or treatment is going to help them feel better. Some children even feel they are being punished or have done something terribly wrong when they are ill.

Children, like all human beings, fear what they do not know or understand. Even the smallest procedure seems major. Parents, adults, and health care professionals who take the time to explain what is happening and to increase a child's knowledge are apt to have a soothing effect and reduce some anxiety.

A health care professional should consider the relationship between children and the parents or primary caregivers. A good relationship with them will lessen the problems with their children.

To respond to children therapeutically, there are several guidelines to keep in mind.

The environment is important for children. Pediatric offices should be colorful, attractive, and comfortable. There should be safe and clean toys for infants and children to keep their minds active and distracted from procedures.

The health professional should establish a friendly relationship with each child. This is accomplished by focusing attention on the child. Kneel in front of children, make eye contact and speak directly to them on their level of understanding. You might mention something positive about the shirt or shoes they are wearing or ask something about the teddy bear they are holding. A positive approach, praise for accomplishments, and acknowledgment of desirable behaviors is much more effective than negative or critical approaches.

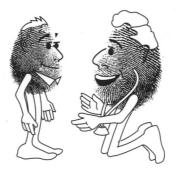

"I really like the shirt you're wearing today."

Infants should be held lovingly for a few minutes on each visit, and especially after every painful procedure. They are sensitive to touch and need warmth and love. This will help the infant associate the health care professional with feelings other than pain.

Give a child a choice only when you know the decision will be the correct one. For example, "Shall we see how tall you are first or how much you weigh?" It makes no difference which choice is made, both procedures will be accomplished. Let children help with procedures if you can, but do not lose control of the situation. Johnny may hold the tape while you apply the bandage to his leg.

Do not keep children and their parents waiting. They become anxious quickly. Visits to the doctor's office that are short, have some pleasant experiences, and have friendly, caring health professionals whom children recognize are the most effective.

Help children deal with their feelings. When children ask questions, respond in short, simple answers. Be truthful and honest. Children who become angry and frustrated can hit a doll, pound clay, or draw pictures. Do not expect to be rewarded by children for the examination, especially anything painful. In fact, children may tell you they do not like you.

Listen to the feelings children express verbally or nonverbally. Learn as much about your pediatric clients as you can from parents. Recognize that crying and silence are pleas for comfort and care as well as anger and frustration.

Be aware of your own feelings when approaching children. They know instantly if you are insecure or do not like them. Children can be "unlovable" when they are frustrated, angry, and in pain. You must be personally able to handle their feelings.

Listen to parents' concerns. Respond truthfully, even if the facts may be upsetting. Help parents deal with their children's feeling and behavior. Encourage them to reinforce with warmth and tenderness rather than fear and anxiety.

Give rewards. They can be simple. A hug, even a handshake are good. Children especially enjoy balloons, stickers, and hand stamps. One pediatric office is known by children as the office of "stamps"—they have over fifty to choose from. At the end of each visit a child selects two—one to be stamped on each hand.

Working with children is a challenge, but one that fortunately many dedicated health care professionals enjoy. Keep in mind these guidelines and remember to always enjoy your profession.

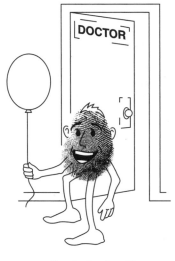

"Look what I got!"

Adolescents

Taking Jeff to the pediatrician as a teenager was different from when he was younger. As they were driving there, Jeff's Mom asked if he would prefer to see the doctor alone. Jeff's immediate response was "Yes." His mom assured him that she was there if he needed her. When they arrived, Jeff quickly picked up one of the car magazines that the office staff had available and promptly ignored the two children playing the child's corner.

When Jeff was called in, he proudly marched to the examination room. During the examination, the physician posed a question that he always asked of teenagers. "Jeff, are you sexually active?" Jeff, a little embarrassed, responded negatively, but the physician hastened on. "It is a question I ask all my teenagers, and I'll ask you when you are in next year. It is important for me to have a truthful answer. It is good you are not yet sexually active. Girls are wonderful; sex is wonderful; but both are addicting." Jeff laughed. The ice had been broken for future discussions regarding sex.

———

Adolescence is a period of transition from childhood to adolescent. Adolescents fight for their independence yet have the same needs for comfort and security as children. It is a turbulent time for teenagers as well as their parents and primary caregivers.

Many demands are placed on adolescents. The demands come from family, school, peers, and society. The bodies of adolescents are changing. They are awkward and feel unsure of themselves. They are confused by their sexual feelings. It is a time when it is vitally important that the adolescent have something to feel good about.

The problems adolescents face often seem insurmountable to them. They may suffer from unsightly acne. Many girls have painful menstruation. Boys may begin to have nocturnal emissions. There is an enormous amount of pressure from peers, who often have misguided notion or fantasy of what an adolescent is expected to be.

Another reason this is a difficult period is that parents, who are often occupied with earning a living and making a career for themselves and their families, are also perplexed with the sudden changes in their adolescent sons and daughters. Teenagers and their parents are likely to have opposing views on just about everything.

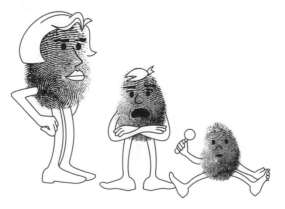

"Why can't I drive?"

Parents may react to their adolescents' attitudes and activities defensively. Parents may feel "put down" by these attitudes and view a rising competition between themselves and their children. Parents can become so anxious themselves that they ridicule and condemn their children in defense of their own insecurities. What adolescents need more than ever during this time is positive reinforcement, encouragement, and understanding.

Some guidelines for responding to adolescents therapeutically include the following.

Allow the adolescent privacy and the right to be examined or treated without parents present. It is best not to moralize, but to generate an atmosphere in which the teenager will feel comfortable to ask questions and seek information.

Do not assume that parents have told their teenagers everything they need to know about sex. Use correct anatomical and socially accepted terms for genitalia and sexual expressions and provide accurate and factual information through books, pamphlets, hotlines, and Web sites. Not only do adolescents need to understand their sexuality physiologically and emotionally, they also must understand safer sex and the responsibility that goes with being sexually active. Health care professionals often avoid this topic, but the events in today's society no longer allow such an attitude.

Treat adolescents with respect and dignity. Ask open-ended questions about their worries and concerns and avoid making comments about their clothes or hairstyle or speaking about good grades as the only important endeavor. Find out what is important in their lives, how they like to spend their time, and what kind of concerns they have. Make notes for their chart so you can bring up the topic at their next visit.

Set limits that are fair and consistent. In this way you can discourage antisocial behavior while encouraging self-control and establishment of identity. Do not take sides in a teenager's battle with parents. Help both parent and teenager assess and understand their positions.

You must clearly like and care about adolescents. If you do not, you will be ineffective in being therapeutic. You cannot hide your feelings from children and adolescents.

Set the stage for the adolescent's transfer from pediatric care to adult care. Young adults often struggle in this transition to establish a relationship with a personal physician. During college years or their first years of employment, young

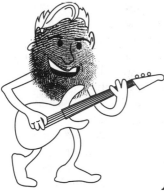

"I like that song, please play it again."

adults are often away from home and have only minimal financial resources. Help instill in their minds the importance of quality medical care throughout their lifetime.

Adolescents need to feel a sense of worth. They need time and understanding to resolve the tensions they feel. The health care professional can be a positive force in this direction. Adolescents welcome established limits that offer security but allow them to gain a little bit of adulthood. Listen to the adolescent; you may be surprised at what you learn.

Adults

As the assistant is recording Karen's vital signs and taking a chief complaint, she asks how everything else is going. Karen relates some difficulty dealing with a teenage daughter who is not doing well in school and whose behavior is troublesome. The assistant responds, "That is quite a worry, isn't it? Your doctor has a lot of skills in helping parents cope with teenagers. Let me mention your concern to him. Also, we have some wonderful pamphlets at the front desk that might help. I'll collect some for you to take home."

Karen is relieved that she will be able to talk with someone about her concerns. She is feeling like such a failure as a parent right now.

———

Many of the principles applied to children and adolescents are appropriate for adults of all ages. Adults should be recognized for the characteristic activities of this age group—working toward life's vocation, earning a living, establishing primary relationships, making a place for themselves in a community, and perhaps raising a family.

Because these activities require an inordinate amount of responsibility, you will find a fair amount of stress-related complaints in this age group. This group also can benefit from information and assistance regarding daily living and parenting. For instance, if a child suffers from a chronic illness, the astute and therapeutic physician recognizes the need to care for the parents also. Education will be an important component of each helping interview.

Younger adults may actually be living in an extended psychological adolescent period since many are still pursuing an education or are not independent from parents.

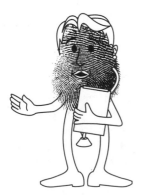

"The doctor said your lab results are all good."

However, the fact that these young adults are physically mature and are most likely living an adult life in all other ways is a source of conflict to be recognized.

Physically, persons in this age group are quite healthy. Women are apt to be bearing children in the younger adult years or facing menopause in their 40s and 50s. Men will pass through a period identified as climacteric when their hormone production tends to slow and diminish.

It is especially crucial during the adult years to recognize the unequal partnership occurring between client and physician and to equalize the relationship as much as possible. Therefore, keep the following recommendations in mind.

Get to know your adult clients. Never allow a therapeutic interview to pass without a discussion of what is happening in the client's life. As much care will be given with an honest discussion of daily occurrences as from a discussion of a particular ailment of chief complaint.

Recognize the skills and intelligence of your clients and do not try to impress them by unnecessary use of your medical nomenclature. Explain in terms your clients will understand and comprehend. Do not, in any way, talk down to your clients. Recognize the client's desire for information and knowledge regarding treatment and care.

Emphasize preventive health care. While most adults see the physician for a "cure" or treatment for an ailment, use that opportunity to educate clients regarding preventive health measures. This is the life stage when prevention can save time and money and lead to better health in the later adult years.

Recognize your role as a member of the health care team. Adults are likely to have more than one primary care physician. Consider the woman who receives care during pregnancy and delivery from an OB/GYN and staff, but still sees a family physician for all other care. This duplication should complement rather than conflict.

Recognize the stress caused by any accident or serious illness in this age group. This is the age identified as the "prime of life." Any serious ailment or accident is apt to be met with anger, denial, and depression. People in this age group do not think about death or disability; they put off such thoughts for the later adult years.

Respect your clients' right to privacy. Clients have a right to expect that the information shared with health care professionals is protected. Adults often reveal information that could compromise their reputation if known to others. Confidentiality must always be preserved.

Encourage your adult clients to hope for the best, but do not promise specific results. Health care professionals cannot predict a sure outcome and should never do so. Promising a cure only destroys the therapeutic relationship if or when the cure does not occur.

Elder Adults

Mr. Levine is 78 years of age. He has just learned that he has prostate cancer and must have radiation treatment. He is confused about what all this means. Using an anatomical picture, the physician shows Mr. Levine where the cancer is located. He tells him that the good news is that the exam showed the cancer was not advanced nor had it spread.

Carefully, treatment is detailed. Mr. Levine asks the physician to write some of this so he will be able to tell his daughter what is happening. The physician complies and tells him what to expect from the treatment. Mr. Levine leaves the office with an appointment to see the radiologist, but not until the assistant has told him to feel free to call any time with an questions he might have.

————

Persons older that 65 are often characterized as elderly. Persons 85 years of age and older, differentiated as "old-old," constitute the fastest growing segment of the United States population. While the proportion of those over 65 has increased by 24 percent since 1960, the proportion of those aged 85 years and older has risen 174 percent.[1]

Older adults experience fewer acute illnesses, however, chronic illness such as hypertension, diabetes, arthritis, and hearing and vision impairment often plague this age group. At the same time, a loss of self-identity and feelings of belonging often occur when a person retires and/or experiences lifestyle changes.

Older persons may look forward to this period as a time of more freedom, a time to pursue activities they never accomplished in their younger years, and a time for fewer obligations. Others may look at this final stage as a time when they no longer feel needed, a time when they become bored and lack the energy to participate in new activities and a time of fear for the loss of personal safety, financial security, and good health.

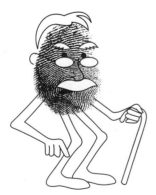

"Some of my parts don't work so good."

The way younger years have been spent is likely the same way the elder years will be spent. If a person has been active and involved, has been a member of one or more organizations, and has had many friends, the same activities usually carry through the elder years. The individual who preferred to be alone, had few interests, and was not a member of any organization generally prefers the same lifestyle in elder years. Some, especially those in business for themselves, find retirement difficult if they have no hobbies or interests.

The elderly population in our society is discriminated against by the popular and always present idea that "youth is better." Models in the media are rarely gray-headed or bald, do not wear glasses, and do not wear half sizes. Another blatant form of discrimination is economic. A large portion of the elderly population live on poverty-level incomes and receive only minimal health care. Even those who are fortunate enough to own a home fear losing it because increased taxes cannot be met by their fixed incomes, which do not keep up with inflation.

All of the guidelines mentioned for a therapeutic response for the adult population should be carried through for elder adults as well. Some additional guidelines are appropriate.

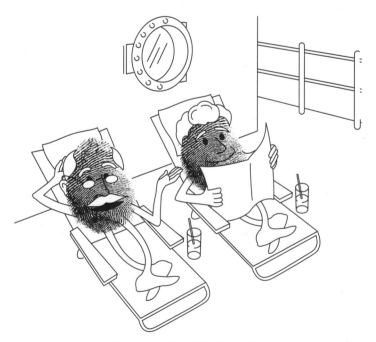

"I'm glad I retired. This is the life."

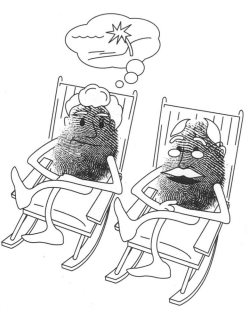

"Too bad we don't have money for that cruise.
Guess we'll have to rock and dream."

Allow additional time for the elder adult to compensate for physiological changes. This client requires more time to ambulate, to disrobe or dress, and may need assistance. More care should be taken in explaining procedures. Talk slowly and clearly. Allow for any sensory deprivation and do not be afraid to raise questions regarding a sensory loss to assess how a client might be better treated. Some are too embarrassed to ask about a hearing loss, for instance, but are relieved when a physician discusses it.

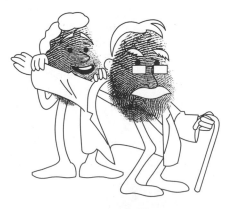

"Let me help you with your coat."

Comfort is important at this age. Be sure your reception room furniture is comfortable. It is easier for older people to rise from a firm, straight-backed chair with arms than from a soft, low sofa. Assess that your examination rooms are adaptable to the elderly. Provide pillows for support and comfort. Handrails in the restroom provide security and support for the elderly and allow them freedom to be autonomous.

A set schedule is often best. The elder adult is comfortable and secure in a routine. Allow for that routine. If a person must be seen weekly to monitor blood pressure, ask that he/she come in on the same day at the same time each week.

Elder person are to be treated with respect and with the recognition that their lives are valuable. Do not operate under the assumption that "since you've lived a full life, you probably won't want to..." Treatment is as important to the older adult as it is to youth. Research has shown that elderly women with breast cancer are not treated as aggressively, on the average, as younger women. Health care providers have made a value judgment about old age.

Do not be oversolicitous or overprotective. This only serves to reduce self-esteem and intensify the feelings the elder adult may be having. With your verbal and nonverbal communication, you can help the client retain self-esteem and confidence during the elder years. Ask what the clients like and dislike about your office and your care of them.

Interest elderly clients in activities as much as possible. A discussion of their daily activities helps to assess if they might benefit from additional activity in their lives. In making suggestions, consider their aptitude, physical abilities, and interests. Be aware of appropriate referrals, such as adult day care, senior citizens' centers, etc.

Help the elderly client remain independent as long as possible. But do not be afraid to honestly indicate when it is time for additional care or altered living situations. Talking with clients to determine what kind of plans they have for the time when they no longer can adequately care for themselves is beneficial in helping clients make their own decisions.

Remember the needs of primary caregivers of the elderly. Whether caring for the elderly in an "at home" environment or in one of the many institutional facilities available today, the primary caregivers must have a respite. A weekend or even a day free of caregiving responsibility is revitalizing and necessary for all parties concerned.

Understand your own feelings toward aging parents or growing older yourself. Try to determine how you would like to be treated and provide the same courtesy to your older clients. The entire staff has the responsibility of helping elder adults feel needed and wanted.

Remember that some diseases/disorders may affect cognition. Cognition refers to processes by which a person knows the world and interacts with it. Cognition involves the way in which the brain learns and interprets information. The human brain is a very delicate and sensitive organ that is susceptible to injury from both internal factors and external factors such as falls causing blows to the head, which may result in brain injury. The use and/or side effects of some drugs, electrolyte imbalance, and ischemia caused by some disease processes are examples of external factors affecting brain function. Therapeutic responses must allow for the cognitive aspect.

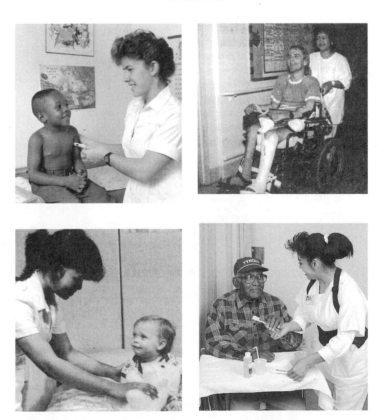

Figure 9-1

Accept each patient in accordance with his or her stage of development.

One of the concepts identified throughout the various age groups is the idea that to be effective in therapeutic communications, health professionals must genuinely like their work and the age groups they are treating. That concept might be applied to any vocation that requires contact with the public as its base. However, dealing with persons who are ill, in pain, and may be dying is quite different than the professional who is making your travel arrangements to go to Paris for a vacation.

Because health care is such serious business, it is even more important for professionals to like their work. Having a healthy respect for life, for each age group and their particular problems, and a mature notion regarding dying and death is a must for effective therapeutic communications. See Figure 9-1.

Exercise 1

In groups of three, identify your personal worst experience in a health care setting. Role-play with a group member how that situation could be turned from your worst experience into one that was therapeutic. Have the third person judge the therapeutic response.

Continue role-playing until each of you has shared the worst experience and identified how to make it therapeutic.

Exercise 2

Interview an elderly person, an adolescent, and an adult. Ask the following questions.

1. When you last visited your physician, how were you treated?
2. What did you like the best?
3. What did you dislike?
4. Why do you seek care from this particular physician?

Exercise 3

Visit a pediatric, children's or hospice wing in a local hospital. Observe the patients' needs and the therapeutic responses offered to these patients by the professionals and paraprofessionals who care for them. Write a brief summary expressing your comfort level with the age group and therapeutic responses you may have offered.

Exercise 4

Search the World Wide Web for information about one or more of the age groups discussed in this chapter. Print out or prepare a list of:

- Telephone numbers and addresses that you might contact for literature
- Internet books, videos, or other media that age groups discussed in this chapter may be interested in researching
- Resources for families needing support information for these age groups
- Chat rooms or bulletin boards for these age groups and their specific needs
- Government Web sites for information on seniors' health care, Medicaid, Medicare, and support groups

Endnote

1. Noreen Cavan Frisch and Lawrence E. Frisch, *Psychiatric Mental Health Nursing*. (Albany, NY: Delmar Publishers, 1998), 527.

Resources

1. Berger, Kathleen Stassen. *The Developing Person through the Life Span*. New York, NY: Worth Publishers, 1998.

2. Frisch, Noreen Cavan, and Lawrence E. Frisch. *Psychiatric Mental Health Nursing*. Albany, NY: Delmar Publishers, 1998.

3. Gamble, Teri Kwal, and Michael W. Gamble. *Contacts Communicating Interpersonally*. Boston: Allyn and Bacon, 1998.

4. Kalman, Natalie, and Claire G. Waughfield. *Mental Health Concepts*, 4th ed. (Albany, NY: Delmar Publishers, 1998).

5. Navarra, Tova, Myron A. Lipkowitz, and John G. Navarra. *Therapeutic Communication*. Thorofare, NJ: Slack, Inc. 1990.

6. Milliken, Mary Elizabeth. *Understanding Human Behavior*, 6th ed. (Albany, NY: Delmar Publishers, 1998).

Chapter 10

The Therapeutic Response to Frightened, Angry, and Aggressive Clients

Procedural Goal

To enhance the student's understanding of therapeutic approaches for the frightened, angry, and aggressive client.

Learning Objectives

Upon completion of this unit, when given a written examination, the student will respond to the following with a minimum of ____% accuracy within the defined class period for the exam.

- Describe the behavior of the frightened client.
- Discuss three therapeutic approaches to the frightened client.
- Describe the angry/aggressive client.
- List at least four descriptors of inappropriate aggressive behavior.
- Discuss at least five therapeutic approaches to the angry/aggressive client.

The therapeutic response implies that the health care professional will be relating to persons in need. Often these persons will be frightened, angry, and even aggressive. Recognizing and understanding such behavior enables the professional to respond in a therapeutic manner.

The Frightened Client

Harry, a 49-year-old construction worker recuperating from a myocardial infarction, returns to the medical office for a follow-up evaluation. Harry is uncooperative; Dr. Cooper discovers that Harry is not taking his anticoagulants, is back to work a month prior to the recommended time, and is still chain smoking. Harry is more concerned during this visit about his sex life than he is about the serious consequences of his behavior.

Fear is an emotion aroused primarily by some sort of threat. Fear of receiving an injection, or having blood drawn are examples of physical fear. Physical fear is usually of short duration; when the experience is over, the fear dissipates. Panic fear on the other hand is an intense fear that may stimulate the person to run from the situation or to be immobilized and numbed by the emotion. The woman who has a family history of breast cancer discovers a lump in her breast and may run immediately to see her physician because of panic fear. If in fact cancer is diagnosed, she may be numb and unable to cope with the situation for a time.

Fright is exhibited in many ways. Physiologically, the client may have sweaty palms, a fast heartbeat, feel a temperature change in the body, and have a sinking feeling in the pit of the stomach. Children exhibit fear easier than adults do. Most adults have been so conditioned by such comments as "There is nothing to be afraid of" that they may hide their fear. Of the adult population, it is even more generally acceptable for a woman to exhibit fear than for a man. This is mostly due to the fact that men have been conditioned to be "brave and strong," showing no fear, and protecting the women around them. Therefore fear is often denied, hidden, masked by other behavior, and eventually turned into somatic symptoms.

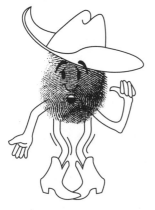

"I'm so scared . . . what if I can't ride my horse?"

The client's denial of fear is an unconscious defense mechanism. Persons using this mechanism will not recognize the cause of their discomfort and may even deny being frightened if someone tells them they look and act frightened. Some clients are so threatened by their illnesses that they will not permit themselves to be aware of their feelings. These clients may become hypercritical of treatment and become unusually demanding. It is difficult for these clients to accept help from their caregivers since to do so is to acknowledge their fear.

Often, frightened clients will not cooperate in their treatment regimen. This is the case in the example given at the beginning of this chapter. For the construction worker to recognize the possible consequences of a myocardial infarction and to take appropriate action is to recognize and accept his fear, also.

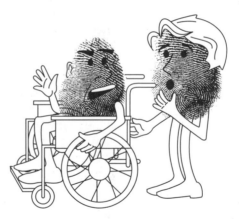

"Buzz off. I can do it."

The Therapeutic Response

Recognize and accept the client's fears. Statements such as, "I know this must be very frightening" can be helpful to the client who feels accepted even though fear has been exhibited.

Use the problem-solving approach. The problem-solving approach often reveals an acceptable solution. Once the patient visualizes a solution, the fear begins to decrease.

Allow the client as much control over the situation as possible. When a client feels in control of the treatment, he/she becomes less fearful. Explain procedures and treatment carefully, taking time to assure and allay the client's fears. This is true even if the client has an extensive medical background.

Act for the client who is panic stricken. Such persons are unable to act for themselves and need the assistance of another. For instance, a person listening to her best friend's panic over a lump in the breast may pick up the phone to make an appointment with a physician for her friend. When panic occurs in the medical office setting, stay with the client until the panic subsides. Explain the situation to a spouse or a friend who may accompany the client.

Panic Attacks

Intense fear, sometimes known as phobias, impact the daily lives of some individuals. Acrophobia is the fear of high places and claustrophobia is fear of being confined in any small space, such as an elevator. Agoraphobia is an overwhelming feeling of anxiety and often leads to a panic attack. Panic attack symptoms may include dyspnea, sweating, vertigo, palpitations, chest pain, nausea, dread, and feeling that there will be a loss of mental control and feeling of approaching death. These fears are abnormal when they interfere with daily living activities or when they cause the individual to take extreme measures to avoid the feared experience. In many cases, it has been determined that some past traumatic experience has been repressed and once revealed and dealt with, the phobia may be managed.

The Angry/Aggressive Client

Janet approaches your desk to make another appointment. She is obviously agitated. She slaps a piece of paper on the counter. You recognize it as a diet the physician has prescribed for her diabetic condition. She sarcastically says to you, "It is impossible to stay on this diet! Who does that doctor think she is?"

––––––––

Anger is another emotion that may be brought on by threats, obstacles or offensive situations. In most cases anger is temporary and is often directed toward a specific object or person. Intense anger directed toward a particular person or persons is termed hate. Annoyance is a term used to describe a very mild form of anger, and resentment is a chronic form of anger that may have a great impact on one's behavior if unresolved after an extended period.

Clients who are angry are easy to recognize. They have an angry tone to their voice and in their facial expression; they are apt to use vulgar language; generally they talk rapidly and rarely listen. Angry clients usually feel frustrated and annoyed. The frustration can come from any number of sources and may or may not be correctly addressed to the health care professional. Janet's frustration may be over a diet she cannot follow because: 1) she likes little or none of the foods, 2) she is afraid that she cannot follow the diet, 3) she is afraid she's losing control over her life, or 4) she's dealing with some totally unrelated incident occurring in her life.

Anger that is not properly managed easily turns into aggression. Every human being experiences these emotions. What is done with the anger and aggression is the key to a healthy mental attitude. Appropriate behavior for these emotions includes physical activity, contact sports, hunting, even watching these activities on television.

Inappropriate expression of anger and aggression includes hostility that is displaced or physically acted out against another person. Hostility is displaced when it is directed toward someone or something other than the cause of the frustration. If a person is angry over circumstances at work and takes it out on the family cat, this is displaced hostility, a defense mechanism.

Helping clients cope with anger and aggression is important. If aggression is turned inward on self, the client may become depressed. Children as well as adults need to be taught appropriate behavior for dealing with their anger.

Some descriptors of persons exhibiting their aggression inappropriately include the following.

- becoming suspicious of others over very small matters
- joking at someone else's expense
- confronting persons with long, involved analyses of their behavior
- becoming hostile, antagonistic, resentful, and carrying a grudge

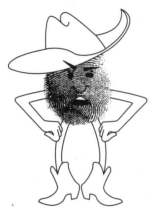

"Who does that doctor think she is?"

- becoming uncooperative, caustic, sarcastic, rude, and critical
- demanding, complaining, and threatening
- threatening to or actually inflicting personal injury

Health care professionals will experience angry and aggressive comments made by clients. To understand and cope with these comments, there are some recommendations to follow.

The Therapeutic Response

Do not take offense at client's comments or take them personally. Evaluate the actions on their merit, not as a personal affront.

A demanding client may really be lonely, anxious, frightened, or insecure. Give reassurance and offer explanations of services or procedures. Try to determine what the client really needs.

Accept clients as they are. Help your clients regain and perceive their self-esteem by talking out their angry feelings. "You seem quite upset about this new diet" is a comment that encourages Janet to tell more about her hostile feelings and does not make her feel ashamed.

Use techniques to deescalate client anger. Speak in a calm voice and use controlled expressions. Let the client know that anger is an appropriate emotion, but that it must be controlled.

Be patient and do not rush interactions. Allow the client to express their anger in a controlled, unhurried atmosphere.

Listen to verbal and nonverbal communication. Remember the communications cycle. You may have to encode the message, check on its validity, and determine the real message. It may be difficult for you to listen. Health care professionals may want to defend their position. However it is best to listen first.

Channel destructive behavior into constructive behavior. Physical activity both as a participant or spectator is beneficial. Pounding a pillow, kneading bread, molding clay, chopping wood, trimming a hedge, or playing the piano or organ are all possible outlets for aggressive energy.

One technique that has been beneficial to many clients is to maintain an anger journal in which the client logs when the anger occurred and what precipitated the anger. It is also helpful for the client to identify how they dealt with the anger.

Document everything. Remember, a deed not documented is a deed not done. Carefully document the entire episode completely.

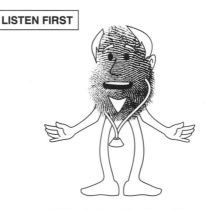

LISTEN FIRST

"Why don't you just listen?"

Clients with severe problems may benefit from psychotherapy. This therapy will help them work through their feelings of aggression and hostility. Recognize when clients require more knowledge and skill than you have and refer them appropriately.

If you find yourself feeling hostile toward clients, you need to examine your feelings and discuss your response with someone who can help you sort through your reaction. Continuous giving to others can drain you and your emotions, but you must be relatively free of anxiety to be therapeutic.

Exercise 1

1. Identify at least three facilities in your community that would be appropriate resources for the client who may be experiencing fear or aggressive behavioral patterns.

2. Discuss with a close friend how you and the members of your living group (family, dormitory roommates, etc.) deal with expressions of anger and aggression.

Exercise 2

Respond to the following situations:

1. Dick, a businessman who has been waiting for his appointment for twenty minutes, says, "I'll not wait another moment for the doctor. Please recommend another physician who can see me."

   Response _____

   _____

2. Sharon, a coworker, remarks to you, "Why do you always insist on making such a mess in the appointment schedule?"

   Response _____

   _____

3. You must tell the client who is smoking in the emergency room that he cannot smoke in the hospital. How will you explain that policy?

   _____

   _____

4. The doctor thrusts a medical chart under your nose and says, "Where are the lab slips that should have been in here a week ago?"

   Response _____

   _____

Resources

1. Frisch, Noreen Cavan, and Lawrence E. Frisch. *Psychiatric Mental Health Nursing.* Albany, NY: Delmar Publishers, 1998.

2. Kalman, Natalie, and Claire Waughfield. *Mental Health Concepts*, 4th ed. Albany: Delmar Publishers, 1998.

3. Milliken, Mary Elizabeth. *Understanding Human Behavior*, 6th ed. Albany, NY: Delmar Publishers, 1998.

Chapter 11

The Therapeutic Response to Stressed and Anxious Clients

Procedural Goal

To enhance the student's understanding of the stress response and how stress affects the human body. Manifestations of stress for each age group will be discussed and therapeutic approaches presented.

Learning Objectives

Upon completion of this unit, when given a written examination, the student will respond to the following with a minimum of _____% *accuracy within the defined class period for the exam.*

- Differentiate between the terms *stress* and *stressor(s)*.
- List five outside agents that may cause stress.
- Describe stress theories as presented by:
  Claude Bernard
  Walter B. Cannon
  Hans Selye
  Thomas H. Holmes and Richard H. Rahe

- Describe the impact of the stress response on the body.
- Identify the four levels of anxiety and describe each.

- Identify signs and symptoms of normal and dysfunctional stress in each age group and list ways to decrease stress for each.
- Identify three therapeutic responses to deal with normal stress and three therapeutic responses to deal with dysfunctional stress for each age group.
- List a minimum of six ways to generally decrease stress.

John and Janice live in a small community and completed a first-aid class several weeks ago. As Janice washed the lunch dishes, she suddenly felt a sense of concern for the safety of her five-year-old son David who was playing in the backyard. Hearing a scream, she ran to the window to see what had happened. Janice felt her heart pounding and her stomach tied in knots. From the window she saw David lying on the ground motionless. He had fallen from the treehouse where he often played.

When Janice reached David's side she noticed how pale he was and his voice was just a whimper. He felt cold and clammy so she quickly removed her sweater and gently placed it around his limp body. Janice called to a neighbor to notify 911, and to bring some water and a washcloth. Janice comforted David and instructed him to lie still. When he asked for water, she gently touched his lips with the wet wash cloth and then placed it on his forehead. David panted for air while Janice continued to speak softly to him and gently smoothed his hair back with her fingertips.

At the emergency room, x-rays revealed a broken leg, which was set and placed in a cast. David spent the night at the hospital for further observation and was discharged the next day.

What is Stress?

The Chinese word for crisis is written by combining two symbols for the word—one symbol meaning danger and the other meaning opportunity. Stress is just that—a danger and an opportunity; a friend and a foe. The term stress has been described as a nonspecific response that requires a person to make some type of change. The body's internal response to change or its adaptive response is termed stress. The demand to change caused by outside influences is called a *stressor.* Stressors cause the body to go into arousal or alarm and may be anything from fear, worry, threatening, or even challenging events. Stressors do not have to actually take place to cause a stress response; just imagining a stress is enough to create a response within the body.

Most think of stress as being something bad or negative and unhealthy. Stress is a normal part of life, it is a useful response, and may be considered positive. We all need a certain amount of stress to keep alive and functioning at peak performance. Too much stress, however, is an enemy and causes the body to malfunction.

During the stress response described in the introduction, Janice felt her heart pound and her stomach knot. Her senses were keen as she quickly assessed David's condition, made decisions, and gave instructions. David's body also responded to the stress alarm. His pale color and cold, clammy skin reflected changes in the circulation of blood. His body made sure his heart and brain had a good supply of blood to ensure survival. The panting kept oxygen levels at their peak.

Stress Theories

Claude Bernard was a nineteenth-century French biologist. He discovered that the body's **internal milieu** (internal environment) changed constantly to meet the daily demands of life. Blood pressure, heart rate, respirations, and the amount of available energy in the circulating blood supply fluctuate to maintain homeostatis. He also learned that if any of these changed too much, the body could not adapt and death followed. One description of "disease" is a condition in which body changes go beyond the limits of normal functioning, though not to the absolute limit the body can tolerate.[1]

Sometimes outside agents such as pathogens, injury and trauma, or environmental pollutants and contaminants cause these changes to the body. Our bodies also have vulnerable spots. Disease and old injuries may leave weak areas that feel the impact of stress. The aging process in general makes us more susceptible to stress symptoms.

A Harvard physiologist, Walter B. Cannon, went a step further than Bernard. Cannon discovered that the body adjusts when change threatens to be too great. For example, when blood is lost through any means, the body compensates for the loss by causing small changes in blood vessels all over the body. The heart rate increases slightly and fluid is transferred from tissues to the bloodstream to bring balance and homeostasis.[2]

Doctor Cannon also discovered that when life-threatening situations arise, excitatory substances are produced. The "wisdom of the body" triggers adjustments causing it to adapt and greatly enhance the body's chances of survival. These substances prepare the body for effort and protect it from harm.

It was Hans Selye who first conceived the theory of non-specific reactions as stress and named his theory *General Adaptation Syndromes (GAS).* Selye theorized that: 1) the adaptive responses a person has are inherited; and 2) these responses vary in individuals. Once the inherited adaptive resources are depleted, the body has no way to produce more. This results in illness, disease, or even death. According to Selye, adaptation to stress occurs in four stages.

Alarm

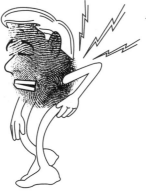

"Ouch!"

This stage is designed to sound a warning when something is perceived to create stress. Pain is a part of this system as it tells us when body tissue is being damaged.

A therapeutic response in the medical office is to recognize the fact that pain does produce a stress response. Ask the client to describe the pain and how it feels. Where is the pain located? Is the pain constant or intermittent? Offer suggestions for coping with pain. Often, breathing in through the nose and exhaling through the mouth will help. If the pain is caused by a procedure in progress, you may be able to distract and engage the person in conversation or reassure the person that it will soon be finished.

Fight or Flight

The sympathetic nervous system prepares the body for fight or flight. The pupils dilate, the mouth becomes dry. The heart rate, pulse and respiration increase. Blood vessels in the skin constrict and blood vessels in the heart and brain dilate. There is decreased motility in the gastrointestinal and genitourinary tracts. All these changes prepare the body for whatever action may need to be taken.

Health care professionals should be alert for these signs and take all measures to decrease the stress response. Recognize that a certain amount of stress will be present no matter why the person is seeing the physician. Provide privacy for those who may be asked to disrobe for an examination. Knock on the door before entering. Keep equipment, instruments, and syringes covered or out of sight. It is very stressful to come into an exam room and see such items and wonder how they will be used.

Exhaustion

The body can only stay in the fight-or-flight state for a limited time. Have you ever stretched a rubber band to the maximum and held it there? After awhile, your body tires of holding the stretched rubber and it is released. When it is released, it has lost some of its elasticity and can never recover it. The same principle applies to the blood vessels throughout the body. After repeated periods of dilation and relaxation, they are weakened. If you have ever overstretched a rubber band you know it snaps. Blood vessels burst when they are dilated to an extreme or have developed weakened areas.

Individuals in this stage may experience physical fatigue. It is best not to give detailed instructions at this time. Rather, allow them to recover—perhaps have them dress after the procedure and relax for a short while. If instructions must be given, it is best to write them out.

Return to Normal

During the return-to-normal stage, the parasympathetic nervous system kicks in and the body returns to normal. The pupils constrict, salivary glands begin to function, heart rate, pulse, and respirations decrease. Blood vessels dilate in the skin and constrict in the heart and brain. The gastrointestinal and genitourinary tracts begin to function again and diarrhea may be experienced.[3]

In the medical setting, these individuals respond well to a calm soft voice. Encourage them to talk about how they are feeling and what helps them cope with the stress. Eye contact and active listening skills will help as well.

All these mechanisms help protect the body and prepare it to escape from danger. However, the body can only stay in this condition for so long. Then the parasympathetic nervous system is activated and the body returns to normal functions again.

Social Readjustment Rating Scale

Doctors Thomas H. Holmes and Richard H. Rahe developed the *Social Readjustment Rating Scale,* which is helpful in charting stressful periods during the life cycle. Most humans experience similar situations that create stress. Whether the experience is positive or negative, we must cope, adapt, or change in some way to meet the demands of the event. Through the use of the Holmes and Rahe chart, it was proven that people tend to get sick or have an accident around the time or shortly after a cluster of major events.

Take time to complete Exercise 1 now.

Anxiety

Stressors affect individuals in different ways. Stressors may be classified as "emotional allergies." We all have them, but they are triggered differently. One of the major responses to stress is anxiety. Anxiety is a feeling of apprehension, worry, uneasiness, or dread frequently accompanied by physical symptoms much as in the fight-or-flight stage. Anxiety is different from fear in that fear is the reaction to a known and usually external threat. Anxiety on the other hand may occur at any time, develops from within, and may be triggered by any situation. There are four levels of anxiety: mild, moderate, severe, and panic.

Mild Anxiety

Mild anxiety is healthy as it increases perception. During mild anxiety, our body functions well. It is stimulated by the increased production of adrenaline, which enables us to think clearly and to focus on details, to be alert, organized and efficient, and to make wise decisions and judgments.

Therapeutic responses to the person experiencing mild anxiety include providing details for health care, instructions, and making decisions regarding treatment.

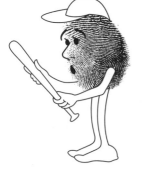

"What if I strike out?"

Moderate Anxiety

The person experiencing moderate anxiety has a decreased perception. The focus is on a particular task or problem rather than on the overall circumstance. This is called selective inattention. When experiencing moderate anxiety, the individual will still be alert and be able to think clearly. Concentration, however, will be focused on one challenge at a time. Decisions and judgments will be made on each individual detail as it is experienced or as the person becomes aware of another detail.

Physiological changes that may be noted during moderate anxiety include perspiration, increased heart and respiratory rates, and muscle tension. Gastrointestinal and urinary tract distress may also be experienced causing frequent urinations and/or diarrhea. Behavioral manifestations may include irritability and pacing.

Therapeutic responses include focusing on one detail at a time, speaking in a soft, calm manner, encouraging relaxed breathing techniques, and keeping the person informed regarding how much longer the procedure will take or the time when the discomfort will be over. Sometimes just saying, "You seem very anxious today" will help the person let go of some of the stress.

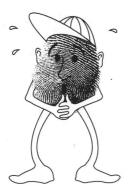

"I don't know what to do."

Severe Anxiety

During severe anxiety, individuals experience inability to focus on details or may be able to focus attention only on one aspect of a situation. Abstract thinking is lost. Some concrete directions may be followed, but learning generally does not take place. Because of the inability to concentrate, these individuals will be very indecisive.

Physiological changes during severe anxiety include dry mouth; profuse sweating; rapid, shallow pulse and respirations; increased blood pressure; headache; speech impairment; increased muscle tension; and tremors or shivering.

Behavioral manifestations include purposeless movements, crying, confused communication, and an inability to think abstractly.

Therapeutic responses to severe anxiety include giving detailed instructions to a family member or writing the instructions for the client. Give them brochures or pamphlets to read after they have had time to gain self-control. Telephone them later in the day or the next day to see how they are doing or if they have any questions.

Panic Anxiety

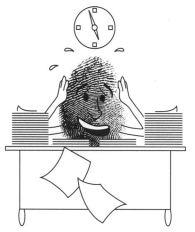

"I'll never finish in time."

During the panic anxiety stage, individuals are consumed with escape. They want to remove themselves from the situation. Attention is focused on a minute detail which is often blown out of proportion. Speech is usually incoherent and communication ineffective.

The physiological changes experienced during the panic stage are the same as the severe stage, only magnified. A prolonged state of panic can cause serious consequences, even death. Behavioral manifestations are also the same as severe-anxiety-stage manifestations only again, greatly magnified.

Therapeutic approaches for panic anxiety are the same as severe anxiety. It is important not to allow a person in this state to leave the office until recovery has taken place or until someone else can drive the person home.

Stress and the Life Cycle

We do not often stop to realize that infants experience stressors, just as older individuals do. Early experiences greatly influence behavior patterns in later life. It is not so much what happens during infancy, but what does not happen that has an impact on behavioral patterns. An infant is totally dependent upon adults for survival. For the infant, the method of expressing stress is to cry. If the stress is not reduced and needs are not met, the only coping mechanism available to the infant is sleep.

To reduce stress, the infant's physical needs must be met. Health care professionals must recognize the fact that not all parents understand or have the basic skills and financial resources to meet these needs. Providing resource information to parents and/or taking some time to teach and instruct is helpful and is more apt to ensure that the infant's needs are met. When parents fail to show interest in the infant and its needs are not satisfied, behavioral patterns are recognizable in the toddler. Often the toddler will display a lack of interest in others and experience decreased communication skills.

Toddlers need consistency. Praise for accomplishments, no matter how small the feat, will build self-confidence and a willingness to keep trying new things. Therapeutic approaches in the medical setting include setting an example for parents to follow in response to the child's development. Many pamphlets, brochures, and books are available to help parents encourage early childhood development. Communication with toddlers is important and interest should be shown in them as individuals. Converse on their level of ability and always remember to be honest with them. If a procedure is going to be uncomfortable and the child asks if it will hurt, explain the process in terms understandable to the child. Tell how it will feel. The injection will hurt like a bee sting or it will feel like a pinch. Toddlers have fantastic memories and will recall if you have been dishonest at one time or another.

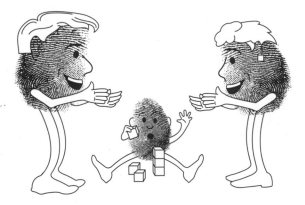

"Good job, Danny. That's a nice tower."

School-age children experience a great deal of stress as they begin the transitional activities between home and school. Suddenly the security of everything known to the child is shaken. When children feel threatened, they often revert to a more infantile behavior called regression. Examples of such behavior include bed-wetting, thumb sucking, or stuttering. Other signals of stress during this time period are nail biting, nightmares, a decreased appetite, headaches, and stomachaches.

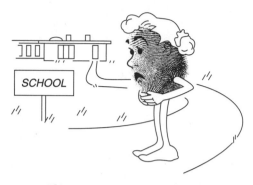

"Oh, my tummy hurts."

To reduce stress for school-age children, suggest that parents discuss the activity well in advance. If possible, suggest a visit to the school, meeting the teacher, taking a ride on a bus, and showing the child where he/she will be met after school.

It is important to be fair and honest with children in the medical setting. Answer questions at their level of understanding and show interest in them as individuals. Never compare one child to another or to a sibling.

Adolescence is defined as a period of change. The body is in the process of changing from child to adult. With these changes comes stress. The development of breasts, narrowing of the waist and widening of the hips, growth of axillary and pubic hair, hormonal changes, and menstruation are some changes females experience. Males begin to broaden through the shoulders and develop upper body strength, facial, axillary, and pubic hair grows. They may experience acne, hormonal changes, and a cracking voice. Growth spurts make them awkward and clumsy.

Adolescents experience social demands and peer pressure as well. They are still children, yet in many ways are considered men or women. They are expected to make decisions regarding college and career goals, and they often begin their search for a mate.

Therapeutic approaches in the medical setting include providing privacy and modesty. Be sure to give plenty of time to disrobe. If possible, provide a drawer, or dressing room closet where their clothes may be placed. Knock before entering the room. Understand that the primary concern of

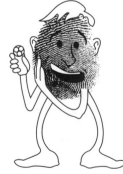

"That's what I call a close shave."

the adolescent is "How will this procedure affect my appearance or level of activity?" Teens fear being different in any way. Be honest and explain the procedure or process in terms they can understand. Respond to their questions and give them choices whenever possible.

Adults experience a variety of stressors. Mortgage payments, career commitments, and perhaps marriage and a family are just a few. Often adults are overloaded with too much to do and not enough time to do it in. Many adults find themselves experiencing the sandwich syndrome. Today's trend is to begin a family later in life with adults becoming first-time parents at the age of 35 or 40. This means their children are still under their roof when they begin to be responsible for aging parents. They are caught in the middle, or sandwiched, between the two generations. Teenagers and aging parents both require intense energy expenditures and create many stressors.

Adults also experience the "empty nest syndrome."

The children are raised and off to college, or married and establishing their own homes. If the children have been the entire focus, the parents may be stressed or depressed.

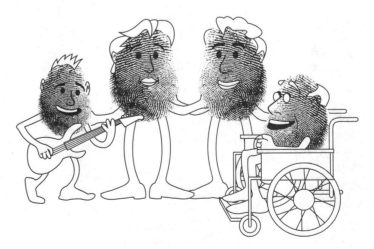

The sandwich generation family

Adults often experience occupational stress or burnout. Some warning signs of burnout include withdrawal from others, negative feelings toward others, increased absences, and less efficient and effective approaches to work-oriented tasks. Irritability toward fellow employees, emotional outbursts, frustrations, and lack of self-control may also be exhibited.

Adults cope with stress better when they have a network of friends and/or colleagues with whom to share. It is always helpful to know that others are experiencing similar feelings and to learn how they are coping with them.

Answer adults' questions in the medical setting. It is often helpful to present pamphlets for details that may be read away from the office setting. Encourage the adult to talk about feelings and fears.

Medical technology has increased life expectancy and today there are many elder adults living useful, healthy lives. Aging is a privilege that provides many past experiences from which to draw.

The elder adult, however, also faces many stressors. Among these are retirement, illness, and death. We think of adolescents experiencing much change during their development. Elder adults also experience much change, and with change comes stress. Much of the elder adults' stress comes from loss rather than gain. They are slowing down physically and mentally. The body deteriorates and wears out. The mind is not as alert and it is difficult to remember the things that were once so important. There is a loss of energy, agility, beauty, and family togetherness. Retirement brings the loss of a job, perhaps security, finances, structure, routine, and relationships. The elder adult experiences the death of friends and acquaintances or even a spouse.

In the medical setting, there are several important steps to take to decrease stress for the elder adult. It is important to answer all questions. Encourage a family member to come along if there is important information to be given or write the instructions for the elder adult. When addressing the elder adult, use the person's full name and title when appropriate. Encourage them to talk about accomplishments and express an interest in the elder person as an individual. Allow the elder adult to make decisions regarding personal health care whenever possible, and use techniques that will foster self-esteem, dignity, and a sense of worth.

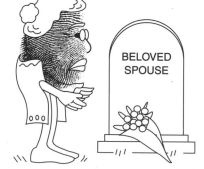

"I've had so many losses lately."

How to Reduce Stress

Reducing stress in your life could have an impact on your overall physical and emotional health. Migraines, high blood pressure, allergies, lower-back pain, depression, and ulcers have all been linked to stress. Here are some suggestions for reducing stress.

1. Any sustained aerobic activity such as running, jogging, or dancing relaxes muscles and also causes the body to release endorphins, naturally produced chemicals that can relieve stress and bring about a sense of well-being.

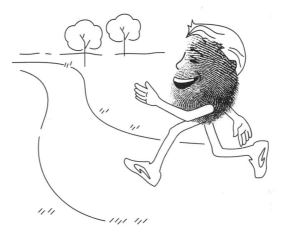

"Jogging really relieves my stress and gives me a new perspective on life."

2. Breathe deeply to feel tranquil. Stress causes quick, shallow breathing that increases tension. By taking deep breaths from the abdomen, you relax and increase oxygen levels to the brain.

3. Take a walk. Whenever possible go outside and walk. Breathe deeply, stand erect, and walk briskly. When high-pressure situations arise in the office or at home, leave the room until you can calm down.

4. Limit caffeine and alcohol. These raise your blood pressure and increase muscle tension.

5. Plan ahead. Whenever possible, rise and shine fifteen minutes earlier in the morning. Get to meetings early and be prepared.

6. Let off steam. When all else fails, let out your feelings privately. Cry into a pillow, punch the couch, stomp your feet, walk, run, or punch a punching bag.

7. Laugh. A hearty laugh is very therapeutic and relieves stress.

8. Nutrition. A balanced diet and regular meals help reduce stress. Too much junk food and unbalanced meals are harmful.

9. Meditate. Silently repeat a favorite word, phrase, or verse.

10. Catnap. Taking a five- or ten-minute nap can rejuvenate and reduce stressed nerves and muscles.

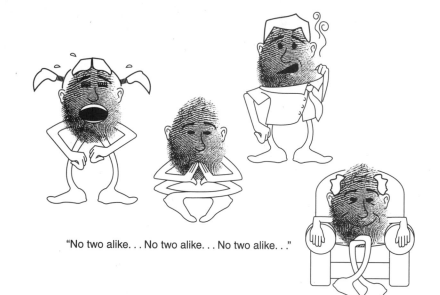

"No two alike. . . No two alike. . . No two alike. . ."

Exercise 1

Using the following Holmes & Rahe's *Social Readjustment Rating Scale*, tally your stress level.

If you scored below 150 points, you are on safe ground—about a one-in-three chance of a serious health change in the next two years.

If you scored between 150 and 300 points, your chances rise to about a 50/50 chance of experiencing a serious health change.

If you scored over 300 points, be sure your health insurance is paid—your chances are almost 90 percent to experience a serious health change in the next two years.

Now list ways you can decrease the stressors you identified. Share this with a friend and discuss.

The Social Readjustment Rating Scale*

	Life Event	Mean Value
1.	Death of spouse	100
2.	Divorce	73
3.	Marital separation	65
4.	Jail term	63
5.	Death of close family member	63
6.	Personal injury or illness	53
7.	Marriage	50
8.	Fired at work	47
9.	Marital reconciliation	45
10.	Retirement	45
11.	Change in health of family member	44
12.	Pregnancy	40
13.	Sex difficulties	39
14.	Gain of new family member	39
15.	Business readjustment	39
16.	Change in financial state	38
17.	Death of a close friend	37
18.	Change to different line of work	36
19.	Change in number of arguments with spouse	35

(continues)

	Life Event	Mean Value
20.	Mortgage over $10,000	31
21.	Foreclosure of mortgage or loan	30
22.	Change in responsibilities at work	29
23.	Son or daughter leaving home	29
24.	Trouble with in-laws	29
25.	Outstanding personal achievement	28
26.	Spouse begin or stop work	26
27.	Begin or end school	26
28.	Change in living conditions	25
29.	Revisions of personal habits	24
30.	Trouble with boss	23
31.	Change in work hours or conditions	20
32.	Change in residence	20
33.	Change in schools	20
34.	Change in recreation	19
35.	Change in church activities	19
36.	Change in social activities	18
37.	Mortgage or loan less than $10,000	17
38.	Change in sleeping habits	16
39.	Change in number of family get-togethers	15
40.	Change in eating habits	15
41.	Vacation	13
42.	Christmas	12
43.	Minor violations of the law	11

*See T. H. Holmes, and R. H. Rahe, "The Social Readjustment Rating Scale," *Journal of Psychosomatic Research* 11: (1967), 213–18 for complete wording of the terms. Pergamon back volumes Microforms International Marketing Corporation.

Exercise 2

Using the Internet, look for self-help, chat rooms, bulletin boards, or other electronic reference sources that could help you, family members, or clients understand and manage stress.

Endnotes

1. Blue Cross and Blue Shield Association, *Stress* XXV, No. 1 (1974); 7.
2. Ibid.
3. Pasquali and Arnold DeBasio, *Mental Health Nursing: A Holistic Approach.* (St. Louis: C. V. Mosby Company, 1989), 233.

Resources

1. Frisch, Noreen Cavan, and Lawrence E. Frisch. *Psychiatric Mental Health Nursing.* Albany: Delmar Publishers, 1998.
2. Kalman, Natalie, and Claire G. Waughfield. *Mental Health Concepts,* 4th ed. (Albany: Delmar Publishers, 1998).
3. Milliken, Mary Elizabeth. *Understanding Human Behavior,* 6th ed. (Albany: Delmar Publishers, 1998).
4. Potter, Patricia A., and Anne G. Perry. *Basic Nursing: Theory and Practice,* 3rd ed. St. Louis: C. V. Mosby Company, 1994.

The Therapeutic Response to Depressed Clients

Procedural Goal

To enhance the student's understanding of depression and depressed individuals, and to identify appropriate therapeutic responses.

Learning Objectives

Upon completion of this unit, when given a written examination, the student will respond to the following with a minimum of _____% accuracy within the defined class period for the exam.

- Define the term *depression.*
- Describe those at risk of experiencing depression.
- List the signs and symptoms of general depression.
- Differentiate between mild and severe depression.
- Describe and list the signs, symptoms and treatment for the following:

  Reactive depression

  Endogenous depression

  Involutional depression

  Manic depression

175

Seasonal affective disorder (SAD)

Postpartum depression

- Identify therapeutic responses to the depressed individual.

Mike lost his job three months ago. He wasn't making much money then, but it was enough to put food on the table for his family. Unemployment will run out in three weeks. There seems to be no hope for another job. The rent is not paid. The recession has hit the area pretty hard; all the plants have closed. Mike is scared. He is very short with the children and appears angry. He has pulled inward and does not talk much. He has no interest in the life going on around him. He has given up hope. Mike is depressed.

Depression accounts for millions of lost production hours annually. Victims usually do not realize they are experiencing depression. Even if they realize the symptoms, they are helpless to fight it. Often, depressed individuals say they have the "blahs," or are experiencing "Monday morning blues." Depression affects the whole body—moods and thoughts, the way we eat and sleep, the way we feel about ourselves and others.

Anyone can experience depression and it can be brought on by a number of different reasons. Signs and symptoms vary, depending upon the type of depression experienced. People may become depressed when their feeling of well-being is challenged or when they experience a loss of some type. Others experience depression because of unpleasant feelings, including sadness, boredom, apathy, even anger.

Depression has been described as feelings of despair, gloom, or emptiness; a sense of foreboding, numbness, hopelessness, or agony; or a negative sense of self-worth. Individuals may look dejected and sad. They may cry for no apparent reason, be quiet with very little to say, and may even shy away from friends and family. Sleeping and eating patterns may be disrupted causing additional fatigue and restlessness.

Mild depression, also known as dysthymia, is manifest by an inability to concentrate, sleeplessness, poor appetite, constipation, amenorrhea, impotence, or disinterest in sex. Individuals may appear unkempt and unshaven. Most depressed persons' thoughts are centered around and related to a loss of self-esteem. They consider themselves losers. Mild depression may or may not have a triggering life event and often occurs for no apparent reason.

Severe or major depression is disabling. Persons have very little desire or energy to do anything. These people become very quiet and do not want to engage in conversation of any kind. They feel inadequate, worthless, and fearful. Persons with severe depression may become incapable of feeling pleasure and sexual arousal, and may stay in bed and not eat for several days at a time. Sufferers of severe depression require professional treatment.

Types of Depression

The four major types of depression are reactive depression, endogenous depression, involutional depression (melancholia), and manic depression (bipolar).

Reactive Depression

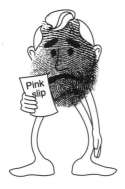

"This is really depressing."

Reactive depression is considered the most temporary form of depression and often follows the loss/death of a family member, a divorce, loss of a job, or not getting an anticipated promotion. *Loss* is the key. The loss may also include the loss of love, beauty, a home—loss of anything with meaning to the individual.

Some signs and symptoms of reactive depression include: 1) a decreased appetite and weight loss of under ten pounds, 2) worsening depression as the day progresses, 3) difficulty falling asleep (DFA), and 4) slowing of body functions, causing urinary retention, constipation, and decreased hormone levels.

Usually individuals suffering from reactive depression are able to work through the emotional distress for themselves. Medications are not recommended since time seems to reduce the situation. Family and friends can be a big support as they may be aware of the precipitating factor. Sympathy and support in a person's time of need help the person resolve what has happened. Showing interest in the person's needs and listening to what is said are extremely therapeutic. Do not become instrusive, however; allow individuals to decide how much, and when, they wish to discuss the situation. Use your best listening skills. As you listen with the ear, observe with the eye any nonverbal communication cues. Encourage individuals to share their feelings. If they cry, remember that tears can be therapeutic, and will help relieve the sadness. Say something like, "I understand how difficult this time is for you. Crying sometimes helps in dealing with a situation."

Endogenous Depression

Endogenous depression comes from within and has no known recognizable source. Endogenous depression is cyclic, meaning that it occurs during particular life cycles or at the same time each year. The middle-age period is the most common life-cycle period and Christmas or springtime are common times of the year for this form of depression. There also seems to be some link to familial tendencies, possibly biochemical in nature.

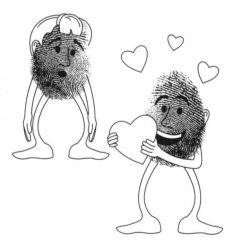

"These special days really make me feel sad and alone."

Symptoms include a substantial weight loss (greater than ten pounds), feeling that the depression came on gradually and out of the blue with no precipitating event. Early morning awakening is often experienced with feelings of worthlessness. However, the symptoms may improve as the day progresses. Endogenous depression tends to be time limited, that is, the depression tends to run its course.

Treatment of the symptoms by use of mood elevators or **tricyclic antidepressants** is the treatment of choice by most physicians. It is important to explain the dosage and any side effects. Many of these medications will change the color of urine. Alert the client to this possibility to avoid adding to the stress level. These drugs also have a lag time, or delayed therapeutic effect. That is, individuals may need to take the medication for up to three weeks before they begin to notice the effects.

Involutional Depression (Melancholia)

Involutional depression usually occurs during middle age or later. Women between the ages of 40 to 55 and men 50 to 65 years of age represent the target group. The personality of individuals who experience involutional depression is often described as rigid, overconscientious, and emotionally unstable. There is usually no previous history of mental illness.

Signs and symptoms of involutional depression include: 1) depression, 2) delusions of sin, guilt, or poverty, 3) obsession with death, and 4) agitation, irritability, and pessimism. The onset of the illness is slow, with an increase in **hypochondriasis** and delusions associated with an exaggerated **paranoid ideation.** These individuals present themselves to health care professionals describing any number of ailments and disorders. Often the symptoms described are subjective, not perceptible to the senses of another person. Negative results of diagnostic evaluations and/or reassurance by physicians only increase the feelings of anxiousness and depression. Individuals become suspicious and mistrust the diagnosis so will seek help from another source.

The prognosis for untreated persons with involutional depression is poor. Treatment with antidepressants or electro-convulsive therapy (ECT)—the use of electric current—has been found effective in this disorder.

Manic Depression (Bipolar)

Manic depression is marked by a series of periods of psychotic depression and periods of excessive well-being. These signs may appear in any sequence and alternate with long periods of relative normalcy. Their mood swings vary in length and may change daily or at longer intervals. Euphoria is the basic effect, with the individual looking happy, unconcerned, and free of worry. These persons usually possess a quick wit and sense of humor. In the manic state, verbal and physical exertion are greatly increased. These persons truly can exhaust themselves to the point where they do not eat or take care of the themselves. Just as those who are depressed neglect themselves in a self-destructive way, manic persons neglect themselves by overactivity in that they have no time for details such as eating, dressing, and organizing time.

Signs and symptoms of manic depression include: 1) inability to converse, 2) a three-second attention span, and a flight of ideas, 3) neologisms and word salads—creating new words by mixing the letters when pronouncing the words, for example, sword walads, 4) hyperactivity, 5) insomnia, 6) minimal self-care, 7) alternating between a sense of euphoria and sadness and apathy, and 8) loss of interest in life.

Lithium carbonate is the treatment of choice for manic depression. There is a very fine line between a toxic dosage and the therapeutic range. Therefore, it is extremely important that blood levels be monitored weekly until they are stabilized. After stabilization, the blood levels should be checked every two months. The blood should be checked the first thing in the morning before medication is taken.

Seasonal Affective Disorder (SAD)

As the winter months progress and daylight hours grow shorter, and winter storms fill the skies with dark clouds, less sunlight is available to brighten the day. These conditions will likely be severe for those who live in the northern parts of the country. The decreased sunlight causes some individuals to develop seasonal affective disorder (SAD).

SAD afflicts about 5 percent of United States adults— some 10 million Americans—but an estimated 25 percent of the population experience some form of winter blues. Winter blues varies in severity from mild "winter blahs," to moderate "winter doldrums," to severe winter depression, medically known as seasonal affective disorder.[1]

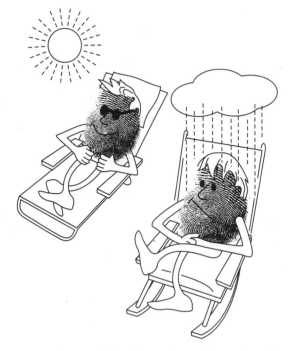

"My get-up-and-go, got-up-and-went."

Women with SAD outnumber men four to one. The disorder also strikes about 4 percent of children and does seem to have familial tendencies. The symptoms of SAD include a noticeable decrease in interests normally pursued during the winter. Some say "my get up and go got up and went." They may experience as much as a 20-pound weight gain during the winter months.

Light therapy or phototherapy has become the treatment of choice for SAD. These individuals should get as much natural sunlight as possible. They may need to trim the bushes around windows or keep curtains and blinds open to allow more light to enter the rooms. They should be encouraged to take walks and consider taking part or all of their vacation during the winter and visit sunny areas of the country. As soon as spring arrives the symptoms disappear.

Postpartum Depression

Postpartum depression is a severe form of "baby blues" lasting anywhere from three months to one year. Stress seems to be one of several contributing factors to this type of depression. A new mother can feel overwhelmed with the responsibilities involved with infants and small children. Sleepless nights, a colicky baby, illness, and lack of physical and emotional support for the new mom all add stress to this new family unit. When one adds the additional factor of fluctuating hormones and their role in postpartum depression, it is little wonder that many women experience this disorder.

Some mothers are afraid to admit they are depressed for fear of being deemed unfit or unable to care for the infant and perhaps losing it to welfare authorities. Support groups can play a major role in recovery. Sometimes just knowing that others also experience similar problems seems to be therapeutic. Physical and emotional support for an entire family can be found in support groups.

Drug therapy can be helpful in some cases; however, caution must be used with the type of medication prescribed. Many medications enter breast milk of nursing mothers and are passed on to their baby.

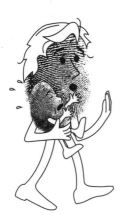

"Why doesn't he sleep more?"

Depression and the Life Cycle

There seems to be no conclusive data to support the incidence of depression in the infant and child. Significant statistics are available to show that the incidence of adolescent depression is greater in females than in males. Factors that increase the risk of depressive responses in adolescents include frequent changes in care takers, changes in family roles, breakup of the home, financial and social strain, death of a parent and the impact on the surviving parent, and the blending of stepfamilies.

Depression often goes undiagnosed in the elder adult. Contributing factors to this oversight may be related to complications brought on by poor health in general, medication interactions, neurological impairment, or the belief that all older persons are normally depressed. Depression is not a normal component of the aging process.

Elderly people do not adapt to change as readily as younger individuals do. Often, the elderly are isolated from family and friends who do not live nearby. The elder person has experienced more loss and grief. Previous coping methods used by individuals will have a direct impact on the individual's ability to adapt and accept change. If you know an elder person who seems depressed, suggest a medical work-up. Reassure them that depression is an illness and is fairly easily treated. Do not delay treatment until the elder person begins to discuss suicide. Compared with younger people, the elderly talk about killing themselves less, but are more successful at the attempts. Fostering a sense of dignity, self-esteem, and value in the elder adult will go a long way in preventing depression.

Therapeutic Approaches

"No. No"

Individuals experiencing the effects of depression must have an environment in which they feel nonthreatened and secure enough to share their innermost feelings. Health care professionals should reinforce the ability to make personal decisions and problem solve. When appropriate, it is helpful to include family members in the problem-solving process.

It is important to identify situations that arouse feelings related to unmet needs. Discussions that stimulate recall of past experiences and positive outcomes and coping methods are beneficial. Assist individuals in manipulating their environments so that they can effect change. Recognize that helplessness may be a learned response and provide situations in which clients can exert some control over their environments.

In response to behavior that indicates hopelessness, do not become "Suzy Sunshine" and try to talk clients out of their depression. Instead, work with them to develop experiences that will provide them with positive feedback.

Exercise 1

Identify your personal responses when feeling "blue" or "down in the dumps." Are these responses healthy or unhealthy? Do they promote resolution to problems or mask and internalize the problem? This exercise is designed for your use only and need not be shared with others.

Exercise 2

Using the Internet, look for self-help, chat rooms, bulletin boards or other electronic reference sources that could help you, family members, or clients understand and manage depression.

Please note that because Internet sources are of a time-sensitive nature and URL addresses may be changed or deleted, searches should also be conducted by association and/or topic.

Resources

1. http:/www.depression.com/types/types_07_seasonal.htm

2. http:/www.depression.com/types/types_08_postpartum.htm

3. http:/www.depression.com/special/special_03_chronic.htm

4. http:/www.depression.com/types/types_04_major.htm

5. http:/www.depression.com/types/types_03_mild.htm

6. http:/www.depression.com/special/special_02_elderly.htm

7. Milliken, Mary Elizabeth. *Understanding Human Behavior,* 6th ed. (Albany: Delmar Publishers, 1998).

8. Frisch, Noreen Cavan, and Lawrence E. Frisch. *Psychiatric Mental Health Nursing.* Albany: Delmar Publishers, 1998.

Chapter 13

The Therapeutic Response to Suicidal Clients

Procedural Goal

To enhance the student's understanding of suicide and how to be therapeutic to persons contemplating suicide.

Learning Objectives

Upon completion of this unit, when given a written examination, the student will respond to the following with a minimum of _____% accuracy within the defined class period for the exam.

- Identify the high-risk groups for suicide.
- List the steps and stages involved in contemplating suicide.
- Differentiate the verbal and nonverbal messages sent by suicidal persons.
- List criteria used to evaluate suicide potential.
- Identify a minimum of five therapeutic approaches to the suicidal person.

Marlene has made a decision. She has decided that her life is no longer worth living. She is making elaborate plans to end it. She calls her sister, Marti, and makes a date to meet her for a cup of coffee. While they are having coffee, Marlene gives Marti a manilla envelope with some personal belongings in it. When Marti opens it, Marlene comments, "It is just some things I want you to have if anything should happen to me."

Suicide: Statistics & Risk Factors

Suicide is the ultimate response to hopelessness, helplessness, and low self-esteem. Every indication or attempt of suicide should be taken seriously. Completing the act provides the final escape from reality for the depressed person.

Documentation indicates that about 15 percent of the population will suffer from clinical depression at some time during their lifetime and that 30 percent of clinically depressed individuals will attempt suicide; half of them will succeed.

An estimated 300,000 Americans attempt suicide annually, and about 30,000 actually take their own lives. The following current statistics have been identified:

- Suicide is the second leading cause of death among college students.
- Suicide is the third leading cause of death among all those 15 to 24 years old.
- Suicide is the fourth leading cause of death among all those 10 to 14 years old.
- The suicide rate for white males (fifteen to twenty-four years old) has tripled since 1950 while for white females (15 to 24 years old) it has more than doubled.
- The suicide rate for all children (ten to fourteen years old) has more than doubled over the last fifteen years.
- The suicide rate for young black males (fifteen to twenty-four years old) has risen by two-thirds in only the past fifteen years.
- Adolescent males commit suicide more than adolescent females by a ratio of 5:1.[1]
- Older people plan suicide carefully and leave less to chance than younger people. For younger people, it is a cry for help; for older people, it is a way out.

Many suicides occur during holiday seasons. The loss of family ties, feelings of isolation, disappointment, and anticlimactic feelings related to the holiday period all may be contributing factors.

Over half the suicide victims communicate their plans to someone before the attempt. They may use one of three approaches.

1. *Indirect:* "What would you do if I were not here to nag at you?"
2. *Direct:* "I wonder what it feels like to die," or "I wonder how it feels to die."
3. *Coded Verbal Messages:* "I hate autumn—everything is dying."

Coded messages are nonpersonal—it is something else that is dying. Just as nonverbal communication must be read in clusters, so these cues must be considered in the context of other messages.

Warning

Most suicides do not occur without warning. By recognizing the signs that indicate someone may be contemplating suicide, and by taking these signals seriously and responding quickly, most suicides can be prevented.

Know who is at high risk for attempting suicide include:

- *Previous attempts of suicide:* Between 20 and 50 percent of people who kill themselves had previously attempted suicide.
- *Depression:* Most suicidal people are depressed; know the signs and symptoms of depression and encourage treatment plans.
- *Situational risk factors:* Stressful life events such as death of a loved one, recent loss of employment, and divorce are examples of situational risk factors.
- *Contagion:* Exposure to suicide or suicidal behavior by others are demonstrated by teenagers and young adults with suicide clusters.
- *Ready accessibility of firearms:* Death by firearms is the fastest growing method of suicide.

- *Demographics:* Males are three to five times more likely to commit suicide than females. Most suicides occur among persons less than forty years of age; however, the Caucasian elderly population displays the highest rate of suicide.
- *Talking about death or suicide:* Over half of the suicide victims communicate their plans to someone before they follow through.
- *Planning for suicide:* Many victims will give things away, say their good-byes, put personal things in order, pay off debts, prepare a will, and make funeral arrangements.

Four Stages of Contemplating Suicide

The individual contemplating suicide usually goes through the following four stages.

Stage #1

The individual's needs are not being met so he/she becomes frustrated. Anger and hostility develop and the anger turns inward. Respond by trying to help the client identify needs not met and the source of the frustration.

Stage #2

A stress situation becomes unbearable and panic sets in. The individual begins to look for a means of escape or to mobilize help. Be a resource to this client and carefully listen to the client's concern. Try to move back to Stage 1.

Stage #3

In an effort to seek help, the individual will communicate his/her helplessness to someone else. This is the point at which you can make a difference. Respond with care. Listen. Let the person know he/she is not alone. Keep in touch.

Stage #4

The individual then begins the suicidal process. The person cannot help himself/herself. The feeling is that no one else cares so, "I'll end it all!" The person begins to develop a plan to carry out the goal, then makes the preparations to carry out the plan. If under a physician's care for depression, the person may call to have a prescription refilled. Next the person carries out the plan by taking the whole bottle of pills at one time. Intervention may be the only appropriate response.

"For patients who telephone or who come into the Suicide Prevention Center in Los Angeles, at least five steps are designated in the treatment process: (1) Establishment of a relationship—maintain contact and obtain information; (2) identification of and focus on the central problem; (3) evaluation of suicidal potential; (4) assessment of resources and mobilization of outside resources; and (5) formulation and initiation of therapeutic plans. At least ten criteria to evaluate suicidal potential have been developed:

1. Age and sex of individual
2. Suicide plan
3. Precipitating stress and patient's reaction to stress
4. Symptoms
5. Resources
6. Characteristic functioning
7. Communication
8. Reactions to significant others
9. Medical status
10. Prior suicidal behavior[2]

Therapeutic Approaches

Prevention is the only significant intervention. Remember, *every* threat or attempt of suicide is serious. This is a time to sit down, pull in close to the individual and listen. Let the person know you really care, that you are a friend or professional, and that you will not leave or desert him/her. Tears are therapeutic, so cry if it is appropriate and you are sincere. Sometimes there is nothing you can do but sit in silence and perhaps hold that person's hand.

Paul Welter, in his book *How to Help a Friend*[3], offered some therapeutic approaches.

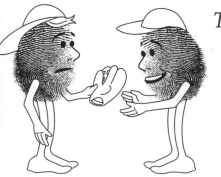

"I really don't use this very much any more and you always liked it. So I'd like you to have it."

1. Listen
2. Do not give "pat answers" and easy advice.
3. Make every effort to understand the mind-set of the person.
4. Communicate through the person's strong learning channel—visual, auditory, or touch/movement.
5. Avoid arguments and power struggles. As a helper, you need to help the person to become less perturbed, not more perturbed.
6. Let yourself feel some of the other person's sufferings, and acknowledge the reality of their sufferings. By responding in an empathic way, you may come across as saying, "I care." This is sometimes an effective way to reduce the amount of self-hatred.

It is helpful to let the person know that you see the pain and agony they are going through and that you care. Encourage the person to talk about how he/she is feeling and why. Ask what you can do to help and be sincere in your offer. Be a resource or link to others who can assist this person.

Have a list of referrals your physician deems appropriate. Discuss with your physician/employer how he/she wishes you to respond in these situations. When in doubt as to your action as a health care professional, ask your physician. Do not wait, though. Time is important in potential suicide.

Exercise 1

Develop a file containing suicide intervention resources for your community. Each resource should include the facility name, address, telephone number, operating hours, specific types of services they offer, fee for service, and any special notes you receive through your interview with the resource.

Exercise 2

Identify the steps you would take if a friend began to send either verbal or nonverbal messages about committing suicide. How would you respond?

Exercise 3

Using the Internet, look for self-help, chat rooms, bulletin boards, or other electronic reference sources that could help you, family members, or clients understand suicide, those at risk, and intervention approaches.

Please note that because Internet resources are of a time-sensitive nature and URL addresses may change or be deleted, searches should also be conducted by association and/or topic.

Endnotes

1. http://www.afsp.org/suicide/whattodo.html; Suicide Facts;
2. Frances Monet Carter Evans, *Psychosocial Nursing* (New York: The Macmillan Company, 1971), 282.
3. Paul Welter, *How to Help a Friend* (Wheaton, IL: Tyndale House Publishers, Inc., 1982), 2811–2812.

Resources

1. http://www.afsp.org/suicide/firearms.htm
2. http://www.afsp.org/suicide/women.htm
3. http://www.depression.com/suicide/suicide_02_ threatening.htm
4. http://www.afsp.org/suicide/danger.html
5. http://www.afsp.org/suicide/children.htm
6. http://www.afsp.org/suicide/facts.html
7. Milliken, Mary Elizabeth. *Understanding Human Behavior*, 6th ed. (Albany, NY: Delmar Publishers, 1998).
8. Frisch, Noreen Cavan, and Lawrence E. Frisch. *Psychiatric Mental Health Nursing.* Albany, NY: Delmar Publishers, 1998.

Chapter 14

The Therapeutic Response to Sexually Suggestive Clients

Procedural Goal

To enhance the student's understanding of therapeutic approaches to the sexually suggestive client.

Learning Objectives

Upon completion of this unit, when given a written examination, the student will respond to the following with a minimum of _____% accuracy within the defined class period for the exam.

- Describe the sexually suggestive client.
- Discuss at least four therapeutic approaches to the sexually suggestive client.

Responding appropriately to the sexually suggestive client is more likely a problem of the physician or a nurse in a hospital setting. Most health care professionals will at one time or another in their careers be confronted with a client who has a sexual problem.

Jerry, a 31-year-old client who was scheduled for an orchidectomy later in the week, was in for an examination. From the moment he entered the office, he began joking about his surgery with the receptionist and medical assistant. He seemed too jovial and unconcerned about the surgery, told jokes with sexual connotations, and tried to make a date with the medical assistant, saying "This might be my last chance."

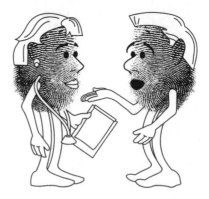

"How about going out with me tonight?"

Attitudes Toward Sexuality

We are all sexual beings. Our feelings and beliefs about sexuality, our ethnic background, our cultural heritage, and our religious experience influence our attitudes regarding sex. Our sexuality includes not only sexual intercourse, but the physical, psychological, emotional, cultural, and spiritual dimensions of sexuality in our lives. We communicate and love through the expression of our sexuality. Our sexuality begins at birth and does not end until death.

Health professionals with a healthy attitude toward their own sexuality will find it easier to be able to respond therapeutically to clients who are having difficulty in expressing theirs. When clients are sexually suggestive, it is usually a result of insecure feelings and a need for reassurance and acceptance. Jerry is not normally so forward in his sexual behavior. He is masking his fear of the surgery and his fear of losing his masculinity. He needs reassurance and acceptance.

Therapeutic Approaches

Some recommendations to follow in dealing with the sexually suggestive clients are provided for you here.

Maintain a positive and healthy personal and professional attitude regarding sexuality. If you have problems or feel uncomfortable with topics that may include masturbation, intercourse outside of marriage, sexual relations between gays and lesbians, and sex change surgery, it may be important for you to seek assistance to help you work through your feelings. To be uncomfortable yourself makes it difficult to respond therapeutically in these situations. It does not mean that you must embrace the behavior; it means that you must understand it and be able to discuss the behavior with your clients in a professional manner.

This may be the most difficult but the most important of the recommendations. The fact that most health care professionals have a difficult time raising *any* discussion of human sexuality with their clients is a sign that most are not comfortable with the topic. To remain uncomfortable and to avoid discussions of human sexuality is to deny a significant part of yourself and of your clients.

Accept the clients for who they are and not for their sexual behavior. Do not be judgmental of their behavior. Recognize your own biases on sexuality.

Be alert for clients' verbal and nonverbal cues for help in dealing with their sexuality. Clients who have an illness or disability that prevents them from engaging in sexual activity must be encouraged to discuss their feelings. Other avenues of expression can be explored.

In a sexual situation, tell clients that you realize they have needs that are normal, but that inappropriate action is not acceptable. With Jerry, the medical assistant might respond, "Jerry, your sexual needs are heightened now because of your pending surgery. These needs are normal, but I feel uncomfortable when you express your needs in this way."

Clients with an altered sexual image need special assurance of their attractiveness. A woman, for instance, who is recovering from a radical mastectomy may feel that the medical staff is repulsed by her altered appearance if they hurry through the dressing change. Maintain eye contact. Do not hurry.

Do not pity, do empathize. Try to put yourself in the position of the client. What might the problems be? What would you want to happen in that situation?

Becoming sexually involved with clients interferes with your goal of being therapeutic and helping clients get well. If there is a genuine two-way attraction, it is your responsibility to acknowledge the attraction but to wait until the client/professional relationship has ended to pursue the relationship.

Exercise 1

Briefly describe what you would say and how you would respond to the individual who is sexually suggestive in the health care setting.

1. The client tells a vulgar, dirty joke.

   I feel ...   I would say ...

2. The client asks you for a date.

   I feel ...   I would say ...

3. The client touches you inappropriately.

   I feel ...   I would say ...

4. The client disrobes or exposes him/herself to you at a time other than during a procedure.

   I feel ...   I would say ...

Resources

1. Hemfelt, Robert, Frank Minirth and Paul Meier. *We Are Driven.* Nashville, TN: Thomas Nelson Publishers, 1991.

2. Schaeffer, Brenda. *Loving Me, Loving You: Balancing Love and Power in a Codependent World.* New York: Hazelden Information Education, 1999.

Chapter 15

The Therapeutic Response to Drug-Dependent Clients

Procedural Goal

To enhance the student's understanding of therapeutic approaches for drug-dependent clients.

Learning Objectives

Upon completion of this unit, when given a written examination, the student will respond to the following with a minimum of _____% accuracy within the defined class period for the exam.

- Describe the drug-dependent client.
- Compare/contrast physical and psychological dependence upon a drug.
- Describe the alcoholic client.
- List the reasons alcoholics usually give for drinking.
- Describe Jellinek's four phases of becoming an alcoholic.
- Discuss a minimum of four therapeutic approaches to the alcoholic client.
- Describe clients who abuse drugs other than alcohol.
- Compare/contrast the use, misuse, and abuse of drugs.
- List the drug classifications most often abused.
- Discuss at least four therapeutic approaches to clients who abuse drugs other than alcohol.

203

Introduction

The abuse of alcohol and other drugs is a major health problem in the United States. Drug-dependent clients are found in every socioeconomic group, with the smallest group being found in skid-row populations in our towns and cities.

The abuse of alcohol and drugs should be treated as a chronic, complex, and progressive disease. However, many people in society, including health care professionals, have a difficult time being as objective in treating a drug-dependent client as they are in treating the client with coronary artery disease.

There are various theories to explain substance abuse. Usually the problem is identified as biological, psychological, and/or cultural. It is probably a combination of all three. Drug-dependent clients usually have low self-esteem, do not tolerate tension or frustration well, have difficulty accepting responsibility for their actions, and often blame others for their problems. Often, they do not believe they have a substance abuse problem.

To further discuss drug dependency, some terms should be defined. Physical dependence or addiction upon a drug implies that clients are so physically dependent upon the drug that to withdraw from it causes physical withdrawal symptoms. Psychological dependence or habituation upon a drug implies a craving for a drug because of the "good feeling" it provides. There are emotional withdrawal symptoms when the drug is abruptly terminated. Drug dependence implies both a physical and a psychological dependence upon a drug. The substance can be alcohol, depressants (of which alcohol is one) and barbiturates, tranquilizers, opiates, stimulants, and/or hallucinogens.

A drug-dependent person is caught in a vicious cycle that begins with excessive use of a drug—disapproval—self-recrimination—guilt—rationalization and denial (defense mechanisms)—and continued excessive use of a drug, as shown in Figure 15-1.

Breaking this cycle is difficult to do but is one of the keys to successful treatment and recovery from drug dependency.

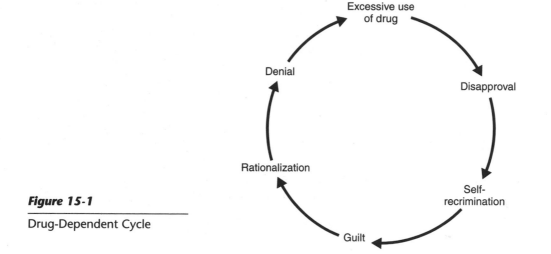

Figure 15-1

Drug-Dependent Cycle

Alcoholism

Jana is a young adult in your medical office receiving prenatal care for her first child. Her pregnancy was confirmed just a few days ago. She seems very frightened and is finally able to tell you that she thinks she is an alcoholic. She begins to cry as she says, "What will this do to my baby?"

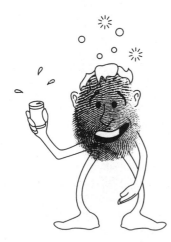

"This feels *good!*"

Alcoholics usually have reasons for drinking: 1) to relieve tension, 2) to relax, 3) to forget about their troubles, and 4) to help them cope with society. The abuse of alcohol interferes with a person's work, family, and social adjustment.

While alcohol can produce a temporary feeling of well-being, it is a depressant (not a stimulant) that acts upon the central nervous system. Intoxication depends upon the amount of alcohol in the bloodstream, with an amount between 0.08 and 0.10 as legally intoxicated. The intoxicated person suffers from impaired vision and poor coordination as a result of the drug's action upon the central nervous system. After the initial euphoria and increased motor activity come clumsiness, staggering gait, nausea, and vomiting. Loss of consciousness, stupor, and coma can occur.

Excessive use of alcohol inflames the gastrointestinal tract, depresses the production of bone marrow, causes both brain tissue changes and scar tissue formations in the liver, depresses metabolism, and reduces an individual's ability to absorb vitamins. E. M. Jellinek has identified four stages or processes to becoming an alcoholic: 1) pre-alcoholic phase, 2) prodromal phase, 3) crucial phase, and 4) chronic phase.[1]

In the pre-alcoholic phase, the occasional drinker begins to drink to avoid problems or to bolster confidence. There is an increase in the individual's ability to tolerate alcohol. The prodromal phase finds a person drinking heavily with the onset of memory blackouts. This person cannot wait to get the first drink, and may gulp it. A fair amount of guilt is felt about the drinking problem, but the person is usually unable to discuss it with anyone. During the crucial phase, there is a loss of control and the person is unable to abstain from drinking. The person exhibits grandiose or aggressive behavior as well as remorse and self-pity while drinking. Withdrawal symptoms will occur if the individual stops drinking. Trouble with family and employer usually occurs in this stage. The chronic phase is marked by periods of prolonged intoxication accompanied by physical and moral deterioration. This person is usually nutritionally deficient. This person is apt to suffer loss of employment and/or divorce and separation from loved ones. If this person is not treated, death may occur as a result of malnutrition, infection, or acute physical problems.

Jellinek stresses the fact that not all phases or symptoms are experienced in every alcoholic, nor do they occur in the same sequence.

Health care professionals are likely to become aware of an alcohol problem while a client is treated for another disorder. Because of the denial problem, few clients readily admit to an alcohol problem or even honestly answer questions related to alcohol consumption during the therapeutic interview.

It is not the purpose of this material to discuss treatment, but it should be stated that treatment will require many facets to be successful. Treatment components include the client's willingness to accept responsibility for the drinking problem, support of family and peers, education about the effects of alcohol on the body, abstinence from alcohol, group or individual therapy, and the support from a group such as Alcoholics Anonymous (AA).

The Therapeutic Response

Health care professionals often have more difficulty maintaining a therapeutic relationship with drug-dependent clients than with others simply because the chance for relapse is so great. It can become depressing to watch a client slip back into the alcoholic state after many months, even years, of sobriety.

Remember that most drug-dependent clients have unresolved emotional problems. Paying close attention to the client's feelings is important in helping to resolve these problems.

Do not moralize or scold clients for their behavior. Everyone else does that to them. They are not able to change their behavior, which is a symptom of the illness. If you have problems dealing with drug-dependent clients, look elsewhere for your employment. If you cannot maintain a therapeutic relationship, you cannot help alleviate the problem.

Help drug-dependent clients set realistic goals for treatment. Encourage discussion, listen carefully, and help them bear the painful feelings they express related to their disease.

Attitudes of compassion, understanding, patience, and acceptance are the best therapeutic approaches to the drug-dependent client. The relationship fosters positive motivation for the client to change behavior. This client needs your strong support but not acceptance of their continued drug dependency.

Involve the family members in the client's treatment plan. Family members and friends need counseling and support, too. Al-Anon and Alateen are groups that can be beneficial for family members and teenagers of the alcoholic.

Refer the client to community groups for continued treatment and follow-up. One of the most popular is Alcoholics Anonymous. Nearly every community has a chapter.

Abuse of Other Drugs

George is 55 years of age. He is determined to stop smoking. His brother just died of lung cancer. George is concerned because he had been smoking two packs of cigarettes a day. It has been a week since George has had a cigarette, but he complains of being agitated, angry with everyone, and unable to sleep at night. He can think of little else other than to smoke another cigarette.

Many clients are drug users. To *use* a drug is to imply that a drug is used according to the directions for medical reasons. To *misuse* a drug implies that directions for the drug are exceeded. The *abuse* of a drug implies that the drug is taken for other than medical reasons.[2] Any drug can be abused. A brief discussion will be made of depressants and barbiturates, tranquilizers, opiates or narcotics, stimulants, and hallucinogens.[3]

Depressants and sedatives or barbiturates have a quieting, sleep-producing effect. Alcohol is the main drug of abuse in this category. Abuse of depressants creates the side effects of slurred speech, impaired judgment and performance, and drowsiness. Their use may lead to shallow respirations, weak rapid pulse, and coma. Withdrawal symptoms include anxiety, insomnia, tremors, and delirium.

Tranquilizers reduce anxiety without producing sleep. Valium may be the most abused in this category. It is often prescribed by physicians for clients who are unable to cope with anxiety and stress. Side effects include fatigue, lethargy, and irregular muscular action. Serious abuse can cause confusion, respiratory depression, and coma. Withdrawal symptoms may not appear until a week or more after discontinuing the tranquilizer and are similar to depressants and sedatives.

The term *narcotics* refers to opium and its derivatives. Heroin, morphine, and codeine are included in this category. Side effects include euphoria, drowsiness, respiratory depression, and constricted pupils. The hazardous effects of these drugs include slow, shallow breathing, clammy skin, convulsions, and brain and liver damage. Symptoms of withdrawal from a narcotic include watery eyes, runny nose, decreased appetite, irritability, tremors, chills and sweats, cramps, and nausea.

Stimulants produce mood elevation and a feeling of boundless energy. Included in this group are cocaine, amphetamines, and nicotine. The side effects include increased pulse and blood pressure, poor appetite, insomnia, and short-term anxiety followed by depression. Hazardous effects include agitation and increased body temperature. The nicotine addict faces the possibility of cancer of the lungs, throat, mouth, or esophagus. Nasal passages are seriously damaged or destroyed by inhaling cocaine. The use of the latter can also result in death from cardiac arrest or ventricular fibrillation. Withdrawal symptoms include apathy, long periods of sleep, irritability, and depression.

Hallucinogens create a sense of unreality and distortion in time, hearing, and vision. Other reactions include hypersensitivity to visual and auditory stimuli. Included in this group of drugs are lysergic acid diethylamide (LSD), marijuana, and phenycyclidine hydrochloride (PCP) or angel dust. As the name implies, hallucinations are induced by these drugs. Hazardous effects include long, intense "trips," "flashbacks," psychosis, and paranoia. There are no known withdrawal symptoms.

A major problem in drug dependency is that many addicts abuse more than one drug. The combinations are dangerous. For instance, alcohol and barbiturates used together can cause death. Persons who abuse drugs may be involved in illegal activity to support their drug habits. Many clients are able to encourage their habits through physicians who carelessly prescribe narcotics and tranquilizers. It is common practice for a drug abuser to have several valid prescriptions for Valium, for instance, which are filled at different pharmacies.

Prevention of prescriptive drug abuse is best controlled by careful assessment of each drug prescribed, careful charting of each refill authorized, and meticulous adherence to the Controlled Substances Act. Potential drugs for abuse should not be prescribed over the phone. Any suspicions the medical office staff might have from such a request should be identified to the physician. Telling such persons that the drug cannot be prescribed without an examination often sends the addict running in the opposite direction.

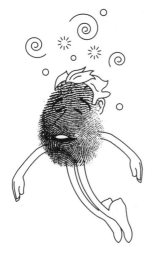

"This is some trip!"

Role of Family and Friends in Drug Dependency

It is important to briefly discuss the role of family members and friends in the treatment of drug dependency. The disease is a problem that affects the entire family. Everyone near the addict suffers. It is not possible or beneficial to try to cajole, beg, or intimidate the drug-dependent person into changing. Alcoholics and drug dependents can only decide for themselves to give up the drugs they abuse. Family members may even become part of the problem when they try to conceal their loved one's problems. This is done by making excuses to employers, giving money when they should not, and generally enabling the drug-dependent person to remain dependent, thereby not facing up to the reality of the problem. There are many support groups dealing with the problem of **codependency** and numerous books written on the subject. Health professionals must also be careful not to become codependent to the problem.

There are five Cs to recall when working with drug dependent clients. They were identified many years ago and have been useful to many who live or work with drug dependency.

Remember:

- I did not CAUSE the disease.
- I cannot CURE the disease.
- I cannot CONTROL the disease or the drug-dependent client.
- And if I try to, I CONTRIBUTE to the problem, and I go CRAZY.

The Therapeutic Response

All the suggestions made for the therapeutic response to the alcoholic apply to any substance abuser. Others to keep in mind include the following.

Educate yourself regarding drug dependency and keep up to date on the latest discoveries. You cannot be therapeutic to a problem you do not understand.

Identify high-risk individuals in your client population. These include children of drug dependents, persons in high-stress jobs, and individuals who have easy access to drugs.

Manage your own negative feelings regarding substance abuse. Do not be discouraged. Do not believe you can "fix it."

Elicit the cooperation and participation of family members and friends in the treatment. Help them understand the codependency cycle.

Encourage the drug-dependent person to seek treatment. This might include group therapy, psychotherapy, self-help programs, Narcotics Anonymous, and/or methadone maintenance programs.

Be tolerant of the client who relapses. Be willing to start again with clients who fail or drop out of treatment.

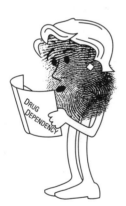

"It says here . . ."

The most frustrating experience when treating drug-dependent persons may be the number of times you will watch clients revert to their addictive behavior. Do not become discouraged or "wash your hands" of the problem. Keep on and encourage the client to reenter treatment.

Exercise 1

1. Identify the characteristics of a drug-dependent person. List the therapeutic approaches for communicating with this individual.

2. Interview a recovering alcoholic or drug addict. Determine what this person's greatest problems are/were. What was helpful? Were there any health care professionals who are/were therapeutic? If so, how?

3. Attend an AA or Al-Anon meeting. Write a brief report identifying your reactions.

Endnotes

1. David J. Pittman, *Society, Culture and Drinking Patterns* (New York: John Wiley & Sons, 1962), 356–68.

2. Natalie Kalman and Claire Waughfield, *Mental Health Concepts,* 3rd ed. (Albany, NY: Delmar Publishers, 1993), 241.

3. Pasquali and Arnold DeBasio, *Mental Health Nursing: A Holistic Approach* (St. Louis: C. V. Mosby Company, 1989), 588–89.

Resources

1. Rotgers, F., D. Keller, and J. Morgenstern. *Treating Substance Abuse, Theory and Technique.* New York: The Guilford Press, 1996.

Chapter 16

The Therapeutic Response to Abusive and Abused Clients

Procedural Goal

To enhance the student's understanding of abuse, abused persons, and abusers and to identify therapeutic responses to abused persons.

Learning Objectives

Upon completion of this unit, when given a written examination, the student will respond to the following with a minimum of _____% accuracy within the defined class period for the exam.

- Describe three types of abuse.
- List at least four characteristics of an abuser.
- Discuss the phases of violence as identified by DeBasio.
- Define:
  criminal violence
  domestic violence
  spousal abuse
  child abuse and neglect
  elder abuse and neglect
  rape
  sexual abuse

- Describe the three forms of elder abuse.
- Identify the three kinds of rapists.
- List possible signs of physical abuse of adults.
- List possible signs of physical/sexual abuse of children.
- Discuss treatment modalities for abused persons.
- Explain appropriate procedures for reporting abuse.
- Identify appropriate therapeutic responses to abused persons.

Sam was brought to the medical office by his granddaughter and primary caretaker, Rebecca. Rebecca always came with her grandfather, but seemed agitated and nervous on this visit. Sam is suffering from the first stages of senile dementia. In the examination room, as the medical assistant rolls up Sam's sleeve to take his blood pressure, she is able to see large black and blue blotches on his skin. She asks, "Sam, what happened here?" Sam replies in a whisper, "Rebecca hits me when I soil the bed."

Introduction

Abuse may be emotional, physical, or sexual. Abusive behavior may come from strangers, friends and acquaintances, and family members. Behavior is violent when there is intent to do harm. This harm may be in the form of emotional abuse which is at first less obvious than physical or sexual abuse. In general, abuse is usually the result of biological, psychological, social, and cultural factors.

Abusers usually suffer from a low self-esteem, a feeling of powerlessness, and blame others for their actions. They are also angry and frustrated. Without self-esteem, it is difficult to be confident and assertive. Persons with low self-esteem and lack of confidence have a difficult time maintaining close and intimate relationships and often feel threatened. Violence becomes a way to gain power and control over others. It is much easier to blame others for abusive behavior than to accept responsibility for the behavior. Abusers are manipulators and easily rationalize and minimize their abusive behavior. Abuse most often occurs when persons have not been able to control their feelings of frustration and anger. The smallest event can trigger an abusive episode. The persons closest to the abuser at this time will probably become the abuser's target.

Phases of violence have been identified by Pasquali and Arnold DeBasio in their book, *Mental Health Nursing: A Holistic Approach.* The phases provide a basis for understanding the abusive act.

Phases of Violence[1]

Triggering

A stress-producing event precipitates the cycle. The abuser humiliates or threatens the victim. The victim may try to placate the abuser by complying or getting out of the way.

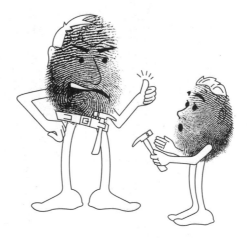

"Can't you do anything right?"

Escalation

The abuser continues to threaten. The abuse escalates as the abuser becomes more enraged and exercises less self-control. There is increased muscle tension, raised pitch and volume of voice, emotional and physical agitation.

Crisis

The abuser loses all control of anger and erupts in physically abusive behavior that may produce serious emotional and/or physical injury, or sometimes death.

Recovery

The assaults decrease as the abuser returns to a baseline level of behavior. In cases of domestic violence and rape, the victim may try to hide, cover the injuries, and/or deny the seriousness of the injuries to self and others.

Postcrisis

Abusers' emotional and physical responses become subnormal. The abuser may apologize and/or use other forms of reconciliatory behavior. A batterer may promise not to be assaultive again and may beg forgiveness. Abusers may sincerely believe that this will be an isolated incident and they will never lose control again.

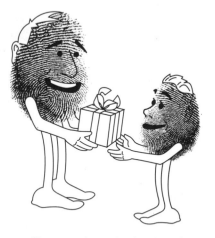

"I'm sorry about what happened.
It won't happen again."

Types of Abuse

Criminal violence exists when a criminal act has been committed. It is not possible in this material to identify all acts considered criminal by each state. Health care professionals must be informed regarding these matters and how they are to be reported.

Criminal violence cannot be predicted. Abusers may have a history of substance abuse, parental deprivation or abuse, and an impulsive personality.

Domestic violence occurs in a family that is dysfunctional. Family violence is seen in all social classes, religions, races, and ethnic groups. In some societies that view family matters as private, outside interference is not tolerated well. Thus, there is a reluctance to report domestic violence.

Spousal abuse refers to abuse between married persons; the abuser may be the female or the male. This abuse also may exist in any intimate relationship even if the couple is not married. The last decade has seen an increase in reports of such abuse. Victims of this type of abuse often report living in relationships characterized by fear, anger, and frustration. Wife battering is most commonly reported, but husband battering is on the rise. Women may receive more serious injuries because generally they have less physical strength than men, but women are more likely than men to use a weapon.

In the United States, women have historically been viewed as property—first of their fathers, then of their husbands. This patriarchal authority is still supported by some cultures and by many organized religions, which may lead some men to believe that if their wives do not submit to their authority, they have a right to discipline them or use them sexually. Abused wives often rationalize that their abuse is caused by their own behavior and their own worthlessness.

It is interesting to note that a person who leaves the abusive relationship or divorces the abuser still mourns the death of the abusive relationship. To obtain emotional health, this individual may need to work through the grieving process.

Child abuse and neglect refer to the deliberate harm or injury of a child by a parent or caretaker. Child neglect refers to lack of care in providing basic necessities to a child. Both physical and emotional child abuse and neglect are evidence of parental frustration, anger, and an inability to fulfill parental obligations.

The term battered child syndrome refers to abused children who are defenseless and unable to communicate the abusive experience. Their sense of self comes from their parents or primary caregivers who are abusing them. This close parent-child relationship often confuses health care professionals trying to make a diagnosis, since both parents and children will exhibit deep concern for each other. Parents bring abused children in for treatment, but are usually careful never to use the same clinic twice and always have an explanation for the injuries. Emotional abuse usually takes its toll in long-lasting physical or psychological problems.

Elder abuse and neglect refers to deliberate harm or injury of an older adult from a personal caregiver. This abuse comes in three forms.[2]

Material

Theft or misuse of money or property for the caregiver's needs rather than the elder's needs.

Physical

Deprivation of medical care, personal care, and/or food; misuse of medications (withholding or overmedicating); battering; misuse of physical restraints.

Psychological

Verbal assaults, threats, and belittling; imposed social or emotional isolation.

Caregivers may be overburdened with the responsibility of caring for an older parent. This may cause the caregiver to ignore the basic needs of the elderly. Often, younger caregivers do not understand the social needs of the elderly. They do not realize that the losses (significant other, driver's license, physical health, etc.) suffered by the elderly precipitate grief. The depression, despair, complaints, and criticism expressed by the elderly who are grieving may become difficult for the caregiver to understand or tolerate.

Psychological and physical changes associated with aging may cause some older persons to withdraw from social activities. Caregivers may tire of sitting and listening to these elderly persons. They assume the role of parent and assign the role of child to the elderly person. This role reversal discourages the older person's independence and integrity.

Rape

Rape is forcible sexual intercourse with an unwilling partner. The rape incident may include **sodomy.** Rape is not a sexual act. It is an act of violence. No person invites rape either by behavior or dress. To say "Anybody dressed like that just asks to be raped" is like saying "Anyone carrying a purse is just asking to be robbed." Health care professionals may find it helpful to recognize that there are three types of rapists: angry, power, and sadistic.[3]

The angry rapist displaces anger on the victim, uses a fair amount of physical force, brutalizes the victim, and degrades the victim by forcing oral sex or masturbation. The angry rapist may even urinate on the victim. The angry rapist most often preys on someone who is older or vulnerable.

The power rapist is the most common type and uses only the amount of force necessary to subdue the victim. The power rapist is seeking power and control and often intimidates the victim. The power rapist may fantasize that the victim is sexually attracted to the rapist, wants to know if the victim "is enjoying this," and may ask to see the victim again after the rape.

The sadistic rapist, the least common type, seeks sexual gratification as an outlet for aggression. Sexuality and aggression go hand in hand. This rapist is aroused by the victim's death, and may achieve orgasm at that moment. Penetration may be obtained with an instrument. The rapist may have intercourse with the victim after death.

Sexual abuse refers to sexual contact between a minor or developmentally immature person and a developmentally mature person. This contact may include fondling, disrobing, showing pornographic pictures, masturbation, sexual intercourse, rape, or sodomy. Such abuse is called incest if it occurs between family members. The incidence of child sexual abuse is not completely known. It is widespread and involves children from every walk of life and at every age.

One in four girls and one in eight boys are sexually assaulted by age 18. More than one-third of the cases involve children under the age of 18. In 80 to 90 percent of the cases, the abuser is known to the child.[4] Child sexual abuse is felt to be the most underreported form of abuse because children often are not believed when they do tell someone. Children may be blamed for the shameful acts or feel too fearful to tell anyone. Often, individuals fail to report cases because they are unwilling to subject the child to questioning or they feel that exposure of a problem may cause more trauma to the child and family than the actual sexual abuse.

People who abuse children sexually often were sexually abused themselves. Abusers may begin to abuse in their teens. If discovered, the excuse of experimentation will often dismiss their offenses. Most sexual abusers will repeat the behavior throughout their lives, even when caught and punished or given treatment. There is certainly no reliable method of changing the behavior of people who sexually abuse children.

Physical Indicators of Abuse

Emotional abuse is not often evident until many years later. However, health care professionals should be aware of those who are often extremely punitive in treatment of others, who are aggressive and verbally abusive to others, and who are easily threatened by others or exhibit a low self-esteem. Victims of abuse typically have few defense mechanisms for coping with anxiety and stress. Health care professionals can and should provide resources for such persons to help them learn to control their abusive behavior.

Physical abuse may be observed by health care professionals when victims seek medical attention or are brought to health care facilities by family or friends. Burns, bruises, lacerations, broken bones, malnutrition—all may be physical evidence of abuse. Special attention should be given to the victim who may deny any form of abuse. It is important to provide victims with information on how to keep safe, help victims realize that they were not the cause of the abuse, and allow them their personal dignity.

Children who are abused will exhibit physical evidence of the abuse. X-rays may reveal fractures in various stages of healing. Burns, bruises, and lacerations are often apparent. Sexual abuse may be evidenced by difficulty in walking or sitting; torn, stained, or bloody underclothing; pain or itching in the genital area; bruises or bleeding in external genitalia, vaginal, anal or mouth areas; and sexually transmitted diseases (especially in preteens) or pregnancy. If medical treatment is sought early enough, rape or sexual intercourse may be evidenced by the presence of semen. In some cases, there may be no obvious physical signs or symptoms.

Children who have an interest in or knowledge of sexual acts or language inappropriate to their age may have been sexually abused. These children may reenact sexual scenes with dolls, in drawing, or with friends. They may attempt to touch the genitals of adults, other children, or animals.

Persons who are physically abused may exhibit aggressive behavior and children also may regress to an earlier stage of development such as wetting or soiling their underwear. Children may threaten their playmates or dolls. Persons may be aggressive toward animals, and anger is directed everywhere. Abused persons often withdraw into a fantasy world. Persons may exhibit fear of specific places or persons. Sleep disturbances and nightmares are common. Nightmares may occur.

Treatment

Physical injuries must receive prompt treatment. The victim needs to have a safe and secure place to go. Provide a list of such places or other possible resources, and discuss alternatives. Focus on the victim, not on the violent event. Underlying anxiety and anger needs to be assessed. The victim needs acceptance and approval and is very vulnerable to any form of rejection, real or perceived.

Eventually, victims must be helped to confront the crisis and talk about their feelings. Victims need to identify effective coping behaviors to deal with the crisis. Community agencies may provide the best resources for this process.

Abusers also need treatment. Health care professionals treating an abuser must be assured of a safe environment for themselves and the abuser. Observing the abuser's personal space is important so as not to appear threatening. A violent person may have a personal space requirement up to four times larger than for a nonviolent person. Involve the abuser in therapy. It is often helpful if the courts require therapy. The abuser must learn assertive, nonviolent ways of expressing anger and frustration and communicating with others. It is best for health care professionals to communicate acceptance of the abuser's feelings but not acceptance of the violent behavior.

Documentation

All states have laws that identify specific requirements for reporting abuse. Each state has laws defining child abuse and mandating that suspected child abuse and neglect be reported. Persons likely required to report suspected abuse and neglect include health care professionals, social service and law enforcement personnel, educators, and professional persons working with children. Any person who believes that a child may be abused or neglected may report, in good faith, to law enforcement or child protection agencies. Such persons are protected against liability as a result of making the report, provided there is reasonable cause to suspect child abuse or neglect.[5] Reports may be made by telephone, in writing, or in person to the local law enforcement agency or appropriate state agency.

It is essential that all information be documented appropriately. Anyone reporting the case should write down the information as clearly and completely as possible. All information is recorded in the medical chart. A brief description of the nature, extent, and location of the injury is necessary. Photographs may be taken to verify injuries. The child protective agencies in your state may have the authority by law to photograph without consent in order to document a child's condition.

The Therapeutic Response

Suggestions are made under "Treatment." However, it is important for health care professionals to examine their own attitudes toward abuse, the abuser, and the victim. Treating abusers with anger and avoidance is not a therapeutic response. Stereotypes about victims of violence need careful self-assessment. Feeling frustrated and powerless to change situations of long-standing abuse may prevent a therapeutic response. A health care professional who has been abused may have difficulty in remaining objective and in being helpful to either the abuser or the abused.

It is important to assist both the abuser and the abused to seek proper counseling. This may involve personal as well as family counseling. Parents Anonymous provides support for parents who have abused their children. VOCAL (Victims of Child Abuse Laws) assists people who have been falsely accused of child abuse. There are support groups for battered persons and rape victims, also.

Unless a trust relationship already exists between health care professionals and the abuser or the abused, it may be difficult to establish therapeutic communication.

It is interesting to note that the victims usually experience the same kinds of feelings as the abuser. Their self-esteem may be seriously damaged by the abusive situation. They feel powerless and often blame themselves. They feel ashamed, frustrated, and angry. They grieve the loss of their self-concept. Significant others and family members pose problems if they are not supportive and accepting of the victim. Health care professionals can assist family members and friends in understanding this dimension of abuse and recovery.

Exercise 1

Select a character who is an abuser or a victim of abuse in a novel, movie, or television program. What kind of behavior characteristics do these persons exhibit? Write a short report with your response.

Exercise 2

Briefly describe what you would say and how you would respond to the following situations. These exercises can be used in small group settings or can be completed independent of others.

1. Your spouse/significant other uses verbal abuse and inappropriate language when you are arguing.

   I feel ...   I would say ...

2. Your date does not listen or respond when you say "No" and "Stop" during hugging, kissing, and fondling.

   I feel ...   I would say ...

3. A stranger approaches who makes suggestive remarks.

   I feel ...   I would say ...

4. You have just been a victim of physical and sexual abuse.

   I feel ...   I would want health care professionals to say ...

Endnotes

1. Pasquali and Arnold DeBasio, *Mental Health Nursing a Holistic Approach* (St. Louis: C. V. Mosby Company, 1989), 633.
2. Ibid., 637.
3. Ibid., 638.
4. Marcia A. Lewis and Carol D. Tamparo, *Medical Law, Ethics, and Bioethics for Ambulatory Care* (Philadelphia: F. A. Davis Co., 1998), 103.
5. Ibid., 103–104.

Resources

1. *Child Abuse.* Washington State Department of Social and Health Services. DSHS 22–174(X), 2/82.
2. *Child Abuse: Guidelines for Intervention by Physicians & Other Health Care Providers.* Washington State Medical Association. Department of Social and Health Services. DSHS 22–285(X), 12/82.
3. Flight, Myrtle R. "Targeting Elder Abuse," *The Professional Medical Assistant* (July/August 1991).
4. *The Facts about Sexual Abuse.* Seattle, WA: A Public Service of Childhaven, A United Way Agency. (Pamphlet)

Chapter 17

The Therapeutic Response to AIDS Clients

Procedural Goal

To enhance the student's understanding of the therapeutic response when caring for persons with HIV infection, AIDS, and AIDS-related illnesses.

Learning Objectives

Upon completion of this unit, when given a written examination, the student will respond to the following with a minimum of _____ percent accuracy within the defined class period for the exam.

- Identify the incidence of HIV infection in the United States.
- Identify the populations in which HIV infection is escalating.
- Describe the HIV.
- Discuss at least four ways persons might become infected with the HIV.
- List at least five realities of AIDS that concern health care professionals.
- Define *AIDSophobia* and discuss its relevance in being therapeutic.

- List at least three challenges for health care professionals in being therapeutic with persons with HIV infection.
- Identify the precautions to take in health care settings to prevent the spread of the HIV.
- Discuss safer sex practices.
- Describe four laws that protect persons with AIDS.
- Identify three ethical concerns in caring for persons with AIDS.
- Identify a minimum of five therapeutic responses to persons with the HIV infection, AIDS, and AIDS-related illnesses.

Chuck waited nervously in his physician's office for his appointment. He was not feeling well. He had a nagging cough, sores in his mouth, and had been losing weight.

His mind flashed quickly over his past. He had left home as a young teen. The drug scene was far more exciting to him than school and basketball. Soon he left the area where he grew up and moved to San Francisco. There he spent more than two years as a male prostitute to support his drug habit.

Chuck was not proud of his past. His mother had never given up on him and stood by him through drug rehabilitation. Although she lived several hundred miles away, they talked on the phone weekly. She had even been supportive of his lifestyle. He'd had an exclusive male partner for five years now. He had a good job in construction and was taking care of himself. If he could only shake this cough, everything would be okay.

Still, the fear was terrible. After many tests yielding no apparent cause for his illness, the physician had suggested that he be tested for the HIV. Chuck would soon have the results.

Introduction

The acquired immunodeficiency syndrome (AIDS) and its related medical problems have emerged as the international health care crisis of the century. In the United States 820,000 people are HIV positive—0.3 percent of the total population.

HIV infection is much higher in poorer nations, however. In some areas along the south Africa border, 70 percent of all adults carry the HIV.

About 16,000 new HIV infections are reported every day. More than 90 percent of these new infections are in developing nations. Children under the age of 15 count for 1,600 of these new cases. Adults make up about 14,000 of the new infections—40 percent are women, and 50 percent are 15- to 24-year-olds.[1]

These shocking statistics come from the U.N. AIDS release of the latest statistics at the 1998 World Conference on AIDS. While AIDS rates plummet in North America and Western Europe where prevention campaigns have proven successful and treatment modalities are more available, the AIDS rates soar in developing nations where death rates have doubled, even tripled in some cases.

Epidemologists are discouraged to discover that groups whose human rights are least respected are the ones most affected. As the epidemic matures within communities and countries, the brunt of the epidemic often shifts from the primary population in which HIV first appeared (gay men) to other populations who are equally socially marginalized or discriminated against (women and children).[2] Just as homosexual and bisexual men are stigmatized by this epidemic, so now are others discriminated against, either because of their gender, race, or economic status.

Those who are discriminated against have limited or no access to prevention information or to health and social services. They are also particularly vulnerable to sexual and other forms of exploitation. For example, the majority of children infected are infected through their mothers during **gestation, parturition,** or through breast feeding. Many of these women do not understand the risk they create for their infants. Moreover, in much of the world, women infected with the virus have low social status, lack of power to insist on safer sex practices, and have no financial means for the recommended treatment protocol.

Researchers predict that the epidemic will continue to slow in industrialized nations, at least for some populations, but it will take a higher toll on socially marginalized groups. The cost of care will continue to rise dramatically as increasing numbers of HIV infected persons receive aggressive therapy.

AIDS is caused by a **retrovirus,** the human immunodeficiency virus (HIV). Viruses are the smallest agents to cause disease in living organisms. They are capable of multiplying only in a living cell. Once inside a host cell, the virus uses the host cell for its own reproduction. The virus undergoes reproduction and maturation. New viruses are produced from the host cell.

The HIV prefers to invade the white blood cells that help defend the body against infection. The immune deficiency caused by the HIV depletes lymphocytes. Without healthy functioning lymphocytes, the immune system collapses, making the body vulnerable to foreign agents. Children are especially vulnerable since their immune systems are still developing.

Everyone is susceptible to HIV infection. No one is entirely resistant. Infected persons do not develop a resistance to the HIV. The HIV is transmitted from one human being to another via fluids—such as blood, blood products, and semen—infected with the virus.

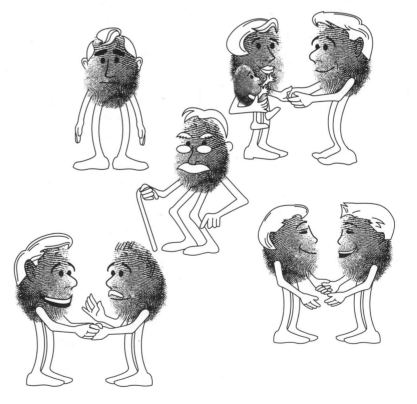

Everyone is susceptible to HIV infection.

People who acquire HIV infection from male-female sex usually have a genital sore through which entry for the HIV is gained. A person with ulcers or erosions of the genital mucosa has several entries for the HIV. Male-male sex may involve anal-receptive sex that injures the delicate lining in the anal canal providing an entry for the HIV.

Intravenous drug abusers who are infected with the HIV and share needles transmit the virus. Since drug abuse is a growing problem in the United States, a higher incidence of HIV infection is evidenced. Persons receiving transfusion of blood products prior to 1985 are at risk for AIDS. Today, however, all blood transfusions are screened and the risk of receiving infected blood is very low. Blood screening for the AIDS virus is not performed, however, in developing nations.

The Realities of AIDS

The infections and malignancies that accompany AIDS can deplete and disfigure the body. The physical weakness and pain resulting from AIDS and AIDS-related diseases compromise a person's ability to cope with stress.

The AIDS virus often attacks the central nervous system, causing symptoms ranging from forgetfulness to profound dementia. The course of the disease is marked by a series of life-threatening episodes, such as infection with Pneumocystis carinii pneumonia.

Few other diseases produce as many losses—loss of physical strength, mental acuity, ability to work, self-sufficiency, social roles, income and savings, housing, and the emotional support of loved ones. Self-esteem usually fades in the wake of such catastrophic losses.

Individuals with no symptoms but who know they have been infected with the virus sometimes are immobilized by fear. Those who belong to the groups at high risk for AIDS face ever-growing problems caused by the public's fear of AIDS as well as the efforts of employers and insurance companies wishing to protect themselves from the economic consequences of caring for persons with AIDS.

Treatment for AIDS and AIDS-related diseases may reduce the intensity and pain but does not cure. The most widely used therapy currently may cost more than $10,000 a year and must be continued indefinitely. Treatment may also cause psychological symptoms of listlessness, depression, and anxiety. Also, medications that may enable *persons with AIDS* to live longer can adversely affect the quality of life as the disease progresses.

The Challenge for Health Care Professionals

When considering all the realities of AIDS just identified, the health care professional is often staggered by the enormity of the challenge of responding therapeutically to the HIV-positive client. Even in the United States there is still a fair amount of stigma attached to anyone who is HIV positive. The immediate question is "How did you become infected?" Individuals are immediately "categorized" by their responses. There is no other life-threatening illness with the same stigma. Health care professionals will want to ensure that they do not carry such discriminatory attitudes into their profession.

Health care professionals also must feel comfortable caring for people who are dying. A special emotional stamina is needed to watch people in the prime of life rapidly deteriorate and die. Spending some time with a **Hospice** group and coming to terms with your own mortality can be helpful.

Many persons with AIDS are abandoned by their families. The only care, concern, touching, and emotional support these individuals receive comes from health care professionals. Meeting these emotional needs can be overwhelming. Health care professionals must have avenues readily available to them to help them cope with such demands.

AIDSophobia is another concern from health care professionals. Even though risk is minimal with proper precautions, some still fear they may contract AIDS while caring for persons with AIDS. Such fears on the part of health care professionals will be evident to persons with AIDS and will block therapeutic communication.

Laws Protecting Persons with AIDS

This material is not designed to be a legal resource for health care professionals. There is wide variance from state to state on legislation, and new laws are being written every day. There are, however, legal recommendations common to all that should be observed.

- Obtain informed consent for HIV testing.
- All information and records containing information about persons who may be infected with HIV must be kept strictly confidential.
- In all fifty states, confirmed cases of AIDS constitute a reportable condition either by statute or administrative regulation.
- Fully comply with your state's requirements regarding the transmission of the disease to others.
- Physicians who are seropositive should consult colleagues as to which activities can be pursued without creating a risk of transmission of the disease to others.
- Expect that persons with AIDS are likely protected under the Americans with Disabilities Act.

The Therapeutic Response

Refer to the next unit on grief, dying, and death for therapeutic responses to persons facing life-threatening illnesses and death. Consider the following suggestions as well.

- AIDS is a disease that elicits moral, ethical, religious, and value-oriented issues. Evaluate your personal value system to determine if it further stigmatizes a population already victimized by society.
- An effective relationship between health care professionals and persons with AIDS can help reduce the alienation, isolation, and rejection often experienced by persons with AIDS.
- Educate family members and significant others about HIV transmission and the course of the disease.
- Provide honest information about the disease and treatment methods in easily understood terms to clients and their significant others.
- Refer to local AIDS service groups.
- Refer to social workers for planning physical and financial assistance.
- Help persons with AIDS learn to live with AIDS and manage their stress.
- Deal with the present, the here and now.

Exercise 1

Determine what support groups are available in your community for persons with AIDS. Select a group, make a phone call to a representative of the group, and discuss how you might volunteer your assistance.

Exercise 2

Log into the Internet and search for sources that provide additional information regarding AIDS and HIV statistics, those at risk, prevention, and treatments. Print out a list of these to share with your classmates.

Endnotes

1. UNAIDS, Laurie Garrett "Newsday," The Seattle Times, 06/24/98, p. A.11

2. Jonathan M. Mann and Daniel J. Mtarantola, "HIV 1998; The Global Picture," *Scientific American,* July, 1998, New York, NY, pp. 82–83.

Resources

1. "Defeating AIDS: What Will It Take?" Special Report from *Scientific American,* New York, NY, p. 81-107.

2. HIV/AIDS Surveillance Report. U.S. Department of Health and Human Services. U.S. HIV and AIDS cases reported through December, 1997. Year-End edition, Vol. 9, No. CDC, Atlanta, Georgia.

Chapter 18

The Therapeutic Response to Clients Experiencing Loss, Grief, Dying, and Death

Procedural Goal

To assist the student in recognizing and understanding the need for a therapeutic response to persons who are grieving and persons who are dying.

Learning Objectives

Upon completion of this unit, when given a written examination, the student will respond to the following with a minimum of _____% accuracy within the defined class period for the exam.

- Describe G.L. Engle's three processes to working through grief.
- Discuss Elisabeth Kübler-Ross's five stages of grief and dying.
- Identify at least six cultural differences in grief and death experiences.
- Identify the five kinds of losses.
- Describe how age factors influence grief.
- Compare/contrast how men and women express grief.
- Explain the difficulties family members have in the grieving process.

- Define anticipatory grief.
- Define dysfunctional and unresolved grief.
- List at least ten losses experienced by someone with a life-threatening illness.
- List at least seven therapeutic responses to grief and death.
- Discuss the impact a Physician's Directive has on dying and death.
- Discuss the steps you taken to face your own death.

Bob felt a sharp and piercing pain in his head, his eyes blurred, and he passed out. Later, after many tests, he learned that he had a benign but inoperable tumor that had spread like a spider web through his brain. Family and friends rallied for Bob's care. Treatment began in the hope of shrinking the tumor.

The night of his death, only a few months later, he told his wife, "I'm going to beat this. I know it is going to be gone when I have my next brain scan." Bob never moved from the denial stage throughout his short illness.

After twenty-one years of seemingly perfect marriage to a minister, Nancy was told that her husband wanted a divorce. Shocked and in disbelief, it was nearly six months before Nancy accepted the fact. It was not until the final papers were signed that she really gave up hope that her husband would return. Her loss was compounded because the church dismissed her husband as their pastor, and she had to leave the home and parsonage she had grown to love. She felt like an outcast.

During grief counseling, she discovered how angry she was and what true rage she was feeling. She learned to release her anger. Without help, she might never have survived the depression without becoming a bitter and very unpleasant person to be around. However, after about eighteen months, her personal fog began to lift.

Slowly, Nancy put her life back together. She changed jobs, began to decorate her apartment with the things she really liked, began to entertain old friends, make new friends, and go on with her life, knowing that the future could be bright. Approximately four years later, she considered herself whole again.

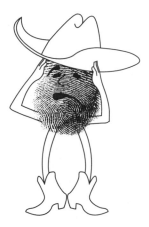

Introduction

Grief, dying, and death are very personal. Dying is a process. Death is an event. Grief is a response. All of us have experienced grief from the loss of someone or something that had great meaning to us. Many, if not all of us, have experienced the death of a significant person in our lives. A few of us may be suffering from a life-threatening illness.

To be therapeutic with persons grieving and dying implies that you have come to terms with your own death. In part, this can be accomplished by gaining knowledge and experience in the grieving and dying process.

G. L. Engle

According to G. L. Engle, one classic theory that provides a solid basis for a better understanding of grief and death identifies three processes to working through grief. They are: 1) *shock and disbelief* that the loss actually occurred, 2) *developing awareness* of the loss and recognizing that it is real, and 3) *acknowledging the loss* in a realistic manner.[1]

During the shock and disbelief process, persons may withdraw from social interaction or have difficulty carrying out normal daily activities. They may also have physical symptoms of sighing, shortness of breath, lack of appetite, and inability to sleep. When persons are finally beginning to realize the loss in the second process, feelings of guilt, anger, and frustration are common. Accepting the loss is the time when persons have a desire to renew their lives and look to the future. They are able to face the loss in a realistic manner.

Kübler-Ross

Another classic theory, that of Elisabeth Kübler-Ross, identifies five stages of grief and loss.[2]

1. *Denial*—This is the time when persons deny reality.
2. *Anger*—This is the time when persons express their anger and rage.
3. *Bargaining*—This is the time when persons are willing to do anything to change what has or is happening to them. ("Let my son live, and I'll change my ways.")

4. *Depression*—Expect deep sorrow and feelings of alone-
   ness when the loss is recognized.
5. *Acceptance*—This is the realistic acknowledgment of the
   loss.

Kübler-Ross first identified this process as stages through
which the dying person might pass. She also learned from her
research that there was no order to the stages and that some
persons never make it through all the stages. In reality, these
stages are now applied to all types of grief and loss. It is also
recognized that persons might pass through all the stages
several times in doing their grief work.

Cultural Influences on Grief and Death

A person's culture and heritage have a significant influence
on the manner in which grief and death are met. Consider
some of the following questions for a better understanding of
culture's role.

Do you place flowers on the grave for the dead person to
smell or do you place tools and food in the grave for the
dead person's journey? Does your culture view death as a
process the entire family embraces or is grief an emotion to
be borne alone? Would you and your family be most comfortable if you died in the hospital or in familiar surroundings
at home? Is the hospital viewed as a place of death or a place
for care and treatment?

Is a health care professional consulted or is a layperson
seen as the most important provider in a time of grief and
death? Is death seen as a punishment from God and suffering viewed as appropriate penance? Is death from violence,
such as murder or suicide, or death from a disease with a
social stigma somehow less socially acceptable than death
from other causes?

Kinds of Losses

Health care professionals will find that there are several
kinds of losses that cause grief. They include: 1) the loss of
personal possessions that have a great deal of meaning, such
as a home destroyed by fire; 2) the loss of a familiar environment, such as a person experiences who must move from an

area especially enjoyed or who loses his/her job; 3) the loss of a significant other in a person's life—life's partner, parent, child, close friend, family pet, etc.; 4) the loss of some part or self—for example, the loss of a limb, the loss of hearing or sight, or even the loss of psychological function such as memory, self-confidence, or respect and love; and finally, 5) the loss of life itself. In the loss of life, the fear is usually not so much from the death itself as it is from the fear of pain and the loss of control over one's life. For some, death is seen as a release or an entry into another life; for others, death and its separation and abandonment are seen as something to fear.

Factors That Influence Grief

A person's age will in part determine how one reacts to grief. *Infants* know only that there is a loss if someone is not there to feed, clothe, hold, and love them. *Toddlers* are confused and cannot distinguish animate from inanimate. Does the chair cry when it is broken? They feel anxious if someone is not there to care for them. *Children aged three to five years* believe that death is reversible. They think the dead person may just be sleeping; they are curious about life and death. *Children aged six to ten years* are very curious about death. Is it cold in the ground? Can the dead move? What happens to the body? They want to do their own funeral ritual. This age group may dig up a dead pet to see what has happened to it. They may feel very guilty about a divorce, blaming themselves and feeling like Mom and Dad do not love them anymore. *Adolescents* have a fascination and a fear about death. They repress and deny feelings and do not talk about the loss in peer groups unless it is the death of one of their own; then they dwell on it. As common as divorce is in the society, adolescents still are devastated by divorce. Adolescents may need help from an older person they care about to cope with their grief. *Adults* sense that loss poses a threat to their pattern of living, perhaps their financial status, but are beginning to examine their own life and its meaning. *Older adults* grieve the aging process, grieve for their friends who have died, and fear a loss of independence.

Men usually have a more difficult time expressing grief openly since they are mostly expected by society to be strong and supportive. *Women* generally have an easier time expressing grief since they are perceived as needing the support of others. The opposite may be closer to truth. It is fairly common in a retirement community for a man to follow his wife in death by only a few months, while a woman may pick up, change her life, and live many years after her husband has died. This may be in part because, traditionally, women throughout their lives are more likely to have a support network of friends to help them deal with their loss. A man more often than not sees his life's partner as the person with whom he can talk and share grief. When that person is no longer present, it is difficult to grieve alone.

It has been said that the greatest grief comes from the loss of a child. Even if a person is 80 years of age and loses a child aged 60, the loss is as great as the loss of a young child. The loss of an unborn infant falls in this category, also.

Everyone grieves at a different rate and in different stages. That is why it is so difficult for family members to help one another. One person may be in denial while the other is in depression; one is angry while the other is in acceptance. It is easy to "blame" the other person for no help or support. It is usually impossible for spouses to help each other in any way other than to share their love and their sadness. For this reason, it is important for family members to seek outside help in their grieving process.

Anticipatory Grief

Anticipatory grief occurs when individuals do part of the grieving process prior to the actual loss. The most difficult grief work usually occurs when the relationship has been one with a fair amount of conflict, ambivalence, and unspoken messages. It is better to spend some time clearing up unfinished business and stating important messages to those close to you before a loss occurs. Many times grief is heightened by the fact that harsh words were spoken during the last encounter prior to death. Anticipatory grief simplifies the grieving process later. Persons with life-threatening illnesses, persons who are dying, persons who know they are going to lose a part of themselves begin the grief process early. This can be beneficial if it helps persons progress to a healthier state after the loss has occurred. It is not beneficial if persons dwell upon the anticipated loss for extended periods.

Dysfunctional and Unresolved Grief

Since everyone grieves at his/her own pace, and because there is really no one "right" way to grieve, caution must be used in labeling unresolved or dysfunctional grief. There are a few considerations to keep in mind, however, that may be helpful. Unresolved and dysfunctional grief can cause unexplained somatic responses, some stress-related medical diseases, and altered relationships with friends and relatives. An inability to cope with loss is disruptive to a person's physiological and psychological functioning. This process may be characterized by uncontrolled crying, hopelessness, helplessness, intense reactions lasting longer than six months, alterations in eating and sleep patterns, denial of loss, idealization of the lost person or object, and a constant reliving of past experiences.

Another kind of unresolved grief may be more difficult to resolve. This kind of grief comes when there is no finish or completion to the death event. A good example is the grief experienced by family members of persons missing in action (MIAs). These people may know only that a body was not found and that their loved one is presumed dead. Crime victims whose bodies are never recovered, victims who are lost at sea—these, too, are examples of death that does not have a final event.

It is often beneficial for grieving family members to establish some kind of completion process. This might include a legal pronouncement of death, a memorial service, or planting a tree in the name of the person who is gone. Even pronouncing that the grief has ended and life is beginning again can be helpful.

Losses Faced by Persons with a Life-Threatening Illness

The term *life-threatening* is used in this writing as opposed to *terminal*. The reason should be obvious, but the use of life-threatening rather than terminal allows a place for hope and empowers a person to a higher degree of control over the circumstances. Persons who are chronically ill, persons who face a life-threatening illness, persons who are dying suffer great losses. They grieve their loss of good health, their independence, their body image, their lifestyle, and their sense of self-confidence (see Figure 18-1). If they may need constant

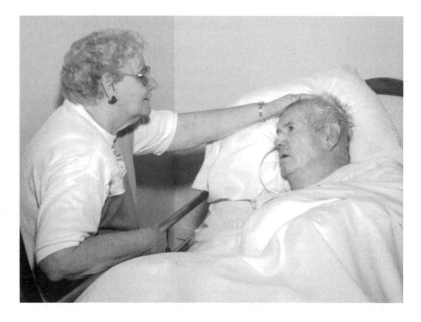

Figure 18-1

The dying person can despair, suppress feelings about approaching death, or reach out to others.

medical care and attention, they grieve their loss of privacy and modesty. Their daily routine is interrupted. Their financial security is usually threatened.

Relationships change. Some are lost; new ones are made. Established work and home roles are radically altered and daily routine is different. Plans for the future may be dashed. It may be impossible to participate in leisure activities once greatly enjoyed.

Sexual functioning may be altered. Sadly, few health care professionals are equipped to discuss this alteration. What is and is not possible with a disability should be discussed. What other forms of sexual expression might be encouraged if sexual intercourse is impossible is a question that needs to be addressed.

It is important to keep persons who suffer from a chronic or a life-threatening illness or are dying as comfortable as possible. Attend to their physical needs, teach them how to safely monitor their medications, provide them as much control as possible, answer their questions honestly, and remember the concerns of family members, also.

The Therapeutic Response

When dealing with persons who are grieving, sensitivity is the key. Sometimes nothing you can do will be helpful; other times you can be very therapeutic. Some general guidelines are suggested to help you.

- Acknowledge individual beliefs and values expressed during grief. Listen. Be aware of nonverbal messages.
- You cannot move a person out of denial. You can only help the person remain as close to reality as possible.
- Do not take any expressed anger personally. Be aware that you may try to avoid individuals who express their anger toward you. Avoidance is a roadblock to communication.
- Do not give false reassurance or avoid discussing any problems that may be uncomfortable but must be addressed.
- Express feelings of hope and cheer when appropriate. These emotions are motivators to avoid feelings of helplessness.
- When death is imminent, your presence may be all that is necessary. Promote dignity and self-esteem whenever possible. Do not pity.
- The words "I'm sorry" or "What can I do to help you?" are usually the only ones appropriate to someone who has suffered a great loss.
- Enable the dying person to remain independent as long as possible.
- Recognize that chronic and life-threatening illnesses take a great deal of energy. Help the individual conserve his/her energy as much as possible.
- As a health care professional, do not view death as a failure. It is a continuum of life.

The Right to Die

No matter in what context grief, dying, and death are discussed today, the topic will always turn to a person's right to die. Advance Directives, now legal in most states, and federal legislation in the Patient Self-Determination Act require health care institutions that receive Medicare and Medicaid reimbursement to establish written policies and procedures on advance directives allowing individuals the right to identify clear choices in their death. At the risk of being too simplistic, there are at least two reasons why the courts and individual state constitutions are embroiled over this issue.

The first reason is that from the very first moment education and training begin, physicians are taught to preserve life. Death may be seen as failure. Allowing persons to die, even when there is no hope for survival, is very difficult, even impossible for some. The second reason is that technology looks at death as another fatal disease to conquer at all costs. Medical technology has advanced much faster than has ethics. Without warning, dying persons often get caught in a system in which technology has ultimate control.

One thing is certainly a result of all the publicity and discussion over an individual's right to die with dignity, to ask that no heroic measures be used, and to even seek assistance with death: persons are now better informed and are likely to have made decisions about their death prior to facing the event. These decisions may even be reduced to writing in a legal document called a Living Will or a Physician's Directive.

Medical office personnel will receive such directives from those persons whom their physicians treat. The directives should be discussed with their physicians and filed in their charts. When a person is hospitalized, a copy of the directive should be sent to the hospital. While the client's wishes should be respected and followed, health care professionals cannot be expected to act unethically or illegally. Any problems should be openly discussed to resolution.

Dying persons and family members may request that attending physicians keep the dying comfortable and free from pain. Some might even request active euthanasia by giving a lethal injection of medication. The latter is more likely to occur when the dying process is slow, painful, debilitating, and renders a person unconscious. While refusing to commit an illegal act, physicians can be therapeutic at such a time by acknowledging and accepting the desperation felt, directing such requests to appropriate sources (such as **Hospice** or the **Hemlock Society**), and facilitating the need to discharge the hospitalized client to the home.

Helping others to die is becoming a hotly contested debate in this country. Often the debate is fueled by those who have watched loved ones suffer immeasurably in their dying. Two states have actively sought legislation to this end, which would protect physicians and loved ones from prosecution should they assist in the dying process. In Oregon where the legislation passed, the decision is still mired in the courts. Washington's proposed legislation did not pass.

Assisted suicide is the term when someone provides the means for a person to end his or her life. Euthanasia is the term when someone intentionally acts to terminate the life of a suffering individual. The Netherlands is the only country that allows both. Interestingly enough, individuals discussing their death choices while well and healthy will often propose such measures; however, the closer one is to death, the greater is the desire to delegate such decision-making to professionals. As medical technology and science advances, the problem of how and when to prolong life will become more complex.

It may be helpful to remember that technology is a tool that does not have to be used. Life is not an idol to be worshipped. There is a time to die. Caring may very well be more important than curing.

In his book *Anatomy of an Illness,* Normal Cousins made this statement:

"Death is not the ultimate tragedy of life. The ultimate tragedy is depersonalization—dying in an alien and sterile area, separated from spiritual nourishment that comes from being able to reach out to a loving hand, separated from desire to experience the things that make life worth living, separated from hope."

Exercise 1

With a friend or classmate, discuss what kinds of choices you would make if you knew you were dying. What kind of medical care would you select? What would be most important to you? Write a brief report identifying your choices.

Exercise 2

Plan your funeral or memorial service. Discuss your choices with family members. Write a brief report describing your service.

Read the obituaries in the local newspaper. Then draft your own as you might see it in the newspaper.

Endnotes

1. Marion Nesbitt Blondis and Barbara E. Jackson, *Nonverbal Communication With Patients* (New York: A Wiley Medical Publication, John Wiley & Sons, 1977), 65.

2. Patricia A. Potter and Anne G. Perry, *Basic Nursing Theory and Practice* (St. Louis: C. V. Mosby Company, 1987), 378.

Resources

1. Backer, Barbara A., Natalie Hannon, and Noreen Russell. *Death and Dying Individuals and Institutions,* 2nd ed. Albany, NY: Delmar Publishers, 1994.

2. Lewis, Marcia A., and Carol D. Tamparo. *Medical Law, Ethics, and Bioethics for Ambulatory Care.* F.A. Davis Company, 1998.

Glossary

AIDSophobia	An abnormal fear of contracting AIDS while caring for a person with the disease.
authoritarian managers	These managers often use domineering positions, such as standing over subordinates, and direct communication approaches.
Babinski reflex	A reflex action of the toes, indicative of abnormalities in the motor control pathways.
classical conditioning	A procedure in which a conditioned stimulus through repeated pairings with an unconditioned stimulus comes to elicit the conditioned response.
Cliché	A trite expression or phrase.
clustering	The grouping of gestures, facial expressions, and postures into nonverbal statements.
codependency	Being a partner in a dependency situation. A codependent lets another person's behavior affect him/her and is obsessed with controlling that person's behavior.
cognitive	The ability of one to think and reason logically and to understand abstract ideas.
conditioned response	A learned response (dogs associate the sound of the bell with food and begin to salivate).
conditioned stimulus	Neutral stimulus to evoke response.
conscience	The part of self that judges the self in terms of values and activity; the superego.
conventional level	Kohlberg's theory that moral behavior is what is accepted and approved by others.
cyberspace	The realm of computer technology used to exchange information and to communicate.
defense mechanisms	Behavior that protects the psyche from guilt, anxiety, or shame.
ego	The psychological force that is in touch with reality and mediates between the id and the superego.
ego-ideal	Corresponds to the child's conceptions of what the parents or primary caregivers consider to be morally good.
ego-integrity	A sense of wholeness and satisfaction.
ego-psychology	The study of self, particularly an individual's self-concept.
erogenous zones	Body areas that provide pleasurable sensations.

exacerbation	Period of time when illness worsens.
generativity	Being concerned with the future of society and the world in general.
gestation	The time from conception to birth.
Hemlock Society	The organization that will provide information to interested persons who wish to have a choice in their death event.
hierarchy	Arranged to a specific order or rank; sequential arrangement.
Homeostasis	State of balance within the internal environment of the body.
Hospice	A lodging or organization that is established for persons who are dying and wish no heroic measures to be taken.
hypochondriasis	Abnormal anxiety and fears regarding one's health.
id	A person's basic animal nature, it is unconscious and amoral.
instrumental conditioning	Learned response through reinforcement.
internal milieu	Internal environment.
Johari Window	Four-paned window illustration of human personality, with each pane representing a segment of self.
kinesics	The systematic study of the body and the use of its static and dynamic position as a means of communication.
Landau reflex	When an infant is held in the prone position, the entire body forms a convex upward arc.
locomotion	Ability to move from one place to another; hitch and pull self for movement.
management by wandering around (MBWA)	These managers wonder about the office observing and recognizing positive performance and discouraging negative behaviors while preserving the self-esteem of the employee.
naturalistic	Refers to circumstances seen as beyond human control.
noctural emission	Involuntary discharge of semen during sleep.
Oedipus	Child identifies with and desires sensual satisfaction from the parent of the opposite sex and views the parent of the same sex as a rival.
operant conditioning	Learned response through reinforcement.
paranoid ideation	Suspicious thinking accompanied by feeling that one is being treated wrongly, mistreated, or judged critically.
participative managers	These managers involve subordinates in decision-making opportunities and encourage open discussions and suggestions for solving problems.
parturition	The act of giving birth.
phallic	Pertaining to penis.
pleasure principle	Immediate gratification or primitive drives; whatever satisfies an impulse is good and whatever blocks or frustrates is bad.
postconventional level	Kohlberg's theory that actions are determined by individual; rights or standards such as the described laws and the United States constitution.

preconventional level	Kohlberg's theory that punishment and reward are understood. To do good is to avoid punishment.
premoral	Before one has a moral code of ethics.
psychosocial crises	Conflicts between a person and society or social institutions.
reality principle	That which exists.
reciprocity	Mutual acceptance.
relativism	Differentiation of right and wrong.
restitution	Punishment and reform.
retrovirus	A member of a family of viruses associated with leukemia and sarcoma.
sanction	The act of a recognized authority confirming an action.
sebaceous glands	Glands that secrete oily or fatty substance.
self-acceptance	Being realistic about oneself and at the same time comfortable with that personal assessment.
self-actualization	Fulfilling one's ultimate potential.
self-analysis	To analyze or examine your own personality, behaviors, and mannerisms.
self-awareness	Being aware of oneself as an individual entity or personality.
sodomy	Anal or oral copulation with another person.
spermatozoa	Male sex cell; sperm.
superego	The moral branch of the personality; the ideal self; strives for perfection.
the electronic age	Period in time that is dominated by using electronic technology to perform a multitude of tasks.
tricyclic antidepressants	Drugs that help increase the concentration impulse-transmitting chemicals between neurons.
unconditioned response	An unlearned response.
unconditioned stimulus	Substance used to produce an unconditioned response.

Index

Note: Boldface numbers indicate illustrations.

abusive & abused clients, 213–226
    abusers, profile of, 214–215
    child abuse/neglect, 213, 217–218
    child sexual abuse, 219–220
    criminal violence, 213, 216–217
    crisis phase of violence, 216
    DeBasio's phases of violence, 213, 215–216
    documentation of abuse, 222
    domestic violence, 213, 217
    elder abuse/neglect, 213, 218
    escalation phase of violence, 215
    incest, 219
    Parents Anonymous, 222
    physical indicators of abuse, 220–221
    postcrisis phase of violence, 216
    rape, 213, 219–220
    recovery phase of violence, 216
    sexual abuse, 213, 219
    spousal abuse, 213, 217
    therapeutic response to abuse, 222–223, 225
    treatment of abuse, 221
    triggering phase of violence, 215
    Victims of Child Abuse Laws (VOCAL), 222
acceptance, in grief response, 240
acknowledging feelings, in helping interviews, 51

active lifestyle, elder adults and therapeutic communication, 138
active vs. passive listening, 37
adolescents and therapeutic communication, 130–133, 142
    asking questions, 130–131
    depression, 182
    grief response, 241
    limits, 132
    privacy, 132
    respect, 132
    sexuality, 132
    stress and anxiety in adolescents, 166–167
    transitioning from pediatric to adult care, 132–133
adults and therapeutic communication, 133–135, 142
    avoiding jargon, 134
    characteristics of various age groups, 127
    depression, 182
    establishing relationships, 134
    grief response, 241
    guidelines for communications, 127
    preventive health care, 134
    privacy, 133–134
    stress and anxiety, 134, 167–168
    team attitude to health care, 134
Advance Directives, 245–246
advice & approval, in helping interviews, 46, 55
age groups and therapeutic communication, 127–145
    adolescents and therapeutic communication, 130–133, 142

adults and therapeutic communication, 133–135, 142

children and therapeutic communication, 143

elder adults and therapeutic communication, 135–139, 142

role-playing exercise, 141

web sites for more information, 144

aggression (see frightened, angry, aggressive clients)

agoraphobia, 150

AIDS clients, 227–236

AIDSophobia, 227, 232

children and AIDS, 229, 230

epidemic nature of AIDS, 229

HIV infection, 227–229

hospice care, 232

laws protecting those with AIDS, 232–233

modes of transmission of AIDS, 231

numbers affected, 228–229

retroviral cause of AIDS, 230

risk factors for AIDS, 230

therapeutic response, 233

treatment of AIDS, 231–232

alarm as response to stress, 160

alcoholism (see also substance-abusing clients), 203, 205–207

codependencies, 210

Jellinek's four phases of alcoholism, 206

role of family and friends in alcoholism, 209–210

anal stage, in psychosexual development, 93–94

Anatomy of an Illness, 247

anger (see also frightened, angry, aggressive clients)

grief response, 239

anticipatory grief, 238, 242

anxiety (see also stressed and anxious clients), 129, 157

attention span, 129

authoritarian leaders, 24, 36

autonomy vs. shame and doubt , in psychoanalytical development theory, 96, 101

Babinski reflex, 100

bargaining, in grief response, 239

behavioral and humanistic development, 115–124

belongingness and love needs, 120

classical conditioning, 116–117

conditioned vs. unconditioned response, 117

esteem needs, 121

hierarchy of needs, 116

homeostasis, 120

instrumental conditioning, 118

Maslow's hierarchy of needs, 119–121, **120**

negative reinforcement, 115, 118

operant conditioning, 118

Pavlov's behavior experiments, 115, 116–117, **116**

positive reinforcement, 115, 118

punishment, 115, 119

safety needs, 120

self-actualization, 121

Skinner's theories on behavior, 115, 118

social learning theory, 119

survival/physiological needs, 120

belittling, contradicting, criticizing, in helping interviews, 46, 56

belongingness and love needs, in Maslow's hierarchy of needs, 120

Bernard, Claude, 157, 159

bipolar disorder depression, 179–180

blind areas of self-perception, Johari window, 12–13

body language (see nonverbal communication)

burnout, 167–168

Cannon, Walter B., 157, 159–160

caregivers to elderly, 138–139

changing the subject, in helping interviews, 46, 57

channels of communication, 23

characteristics of successful therapeutic communicators, 16–17

child abuse/neglect, 213, 217–218

child sexual abuse, 219–220

children and therapeutic communication, 128–130, 143

 AIDS, 229, 230

 choices, 129

 depression, 182

 environment, 128

 grief response, 241

 holding infants, 129

 listening skills, 130

 parents' concerns, 130

 relationship with professional, 128–129

 rewards, 130

 stress and anxiety in children, 164–166

clarifying & validating, in helping interviews, 28, 51

classical conditioning, in behavioral theory, 116–117

clichés & stereotypical responses, in helping interviews, 46, 55

closed questions, in helping interviews, 46, 53, 67

clustering of nonverbal cues, 30

codependencies , in drug abuse, 210

cognitive development, 79–87

 concrete-operations period of development, 82–83

 formal-operations period of development, 83

 four stages of cognitive development, 79

 intuitive stage of development, 82

 observing children, exercise in cognitive development, 84

Piaget's theory of cognitive development, 79

preconceptual stage of development, 82

prepoperational period of development, 82

sensorimotor period of development, 81–82

testing children in cognitive development, 85–86

therapeutic communications and cognitive development, 79

cognitive dysfunction, elder adults and therapeutic communication, 139

cohesiveness in communications, 28

communications skills, 23–43

 active vs. passive listening, 37

 channels of communication, 23

 clarity of communications, 28

 clustering of nonverbal cues, 30

 cohesiveness in communications, 28

 completeness of communications, 28

 conciseness of communications, 28

 courtesy in communications, 28

 cycle of communication, 23, 25–27, **26**

 diverse populations, 24, 34–35

 effectiveness of communication, 23

 feedback from communication, 27

 five Cs of Communication, 23, 28

 foreign languages, 34–35

 gestures & mannerisms, 33, 35

 keys to successful communication, 23, 29–30

 kinesics, 23, 29

 leadership qualities, 24, 36

 listening skills, 24, 36–39

 listening, paraphrasing, and repeating communications, 37, 51–52

 Maslow's Hierarchy of Needs, 36

 message in communications, 26–27

 misinterpreting nonverbal communications, 33–34

modes of communications, 23

nonverbal communication, 23, 29–34, 41

posture & position in communication, 32–33

receiver in communications, 27, **27**

roadblocks to effective communications, 24

sender in communications, 26–27, **27**

team communication, 36

technology and communications, 24, 35–36

territoriality in communication, 31–32, 31, 40

verbal communications, 28

compensation, as defense mechanism, 69, 73

completeness of communications, 28

conciseness of communications, 28

concrete-operations period of development, in cognitive development theory, 82–83

conditioned vs. unconditioned response, in behavioral theory, 117

congruency between verbal and nonverbal message, 29–30

conscience, in psychoanalytical development theory, 91

control factor in successful interview, in helping interviews, 47

conventional level, in moral development theory, 109, 110

courtesy in communications, 28

Cousins, Norman, 247

criminal violence, 213, 216–217

crisis phase of violence, in abuse, 216

criticism, in helping interviews, 56, 57–58

Crosswait, C. Bruce, 28

cultural influences, 7

communication differences, 34–35

grief response, 237, 240

cycle of communication, 23, 25–27, **26**

cycle of substance abuse, 204, **205**

DeBasio, Arnold and Pasquali, 215

defending, in helping interviews, 46, 57

defense mechanisms, 69–76

compensation, 69, 73

denial, 69, 73, 149, **74**

displacement, 69, 72

identification, 69, 73

post-traumatic stress syndrome, 71

projection, 69, 72

rationalization, 69, 74, **74**

regression, 69, 70–71

repression, 69, 71

sublimation, 69, 72

undoing, 69, 73

denial

defense mechanism, 69, 73, 74, 149

grief response, 239

depressants, in drug abuse, 208

depressed clients, 175–186

bipolar disorder depression, 179–180

drug treatment for depression, 179–180

dysthymia (mild depression), 176–177

endogenous depression, 175, 178–179

grief response, 240

hypochondria, 179

involutional depression, 175, 179

life cycle experience of depression, 182–183

manic depression, 175, 179–180

melancholia, 179

mild depression, 176–177

paranoid ideation, 179

postpartum depression, 181–182

reactive depression, 175, 177–178

risk factors for depression, 175

seasonal affective disorder (SAD), 180–181, **181**

severe or major depression, 177

signs and symptoms of depression, 175, 176

therapeutic approaches to depression, 183

web sites for more information, 185

despair, 98, 103

destructive behavior, 152–153

disabilities, 8

displacement, as defense mechanism, 69, 72

documenting behavior, 153

domestic violence, 213, 217

doubts, 96, 101

drug abuse (see also substance-abusing clients), 207–210

codependencies, 210

depressants, 208

hallucinogens, 209

misuse vs. abuse, 208

narcotics, 208

prescriptive drug abuse, 209

role of family and friends in drug abuse, 209–210

stimulants, 208

therapeutic response to drug-abuse, 210

withdrawal symptoms, 208

dying clients (see grieving or dying clients)

dysfunctional grief, 238, 243

dysthymia (mild depression), 176–177

economic influences, 8

educational experience, 8

effectiveness of communication, 23

ego integrity, in psychoanalytical development theory, 98, 103

ego psychology, in psychoanalytical development theory, 95

ego, in psychoanalytical development theory, 89, 90–91

ego-ideal, in psychoanalytical development theory, 91

elder abuse/neglect, 213, 218

elder adults and therapeutic communication, 135–139, 142

active lifestyle, 138

allowing extra time, 137

caregivers to elderly, 138–139

cognitive dysfunction, 139

comfort, 138

depression, 182–183

grief response, 241

independent lifestyles, 138

overprotectiveness, 138

respect and dignity, 138

set schedules, 138

stress and anxiety, 168

electronic media influences, 9

emotional dependency on drugs/alcohol, 204

endogenous depression, 175, 178–179

Engle, G.L., 239

Erickson's stages of psychosocial development, 89, 98–103

Erikson, Eric, 95

erogenous zones, in psychoanalytical development theory, 89, 92

escalation phase of violence, in abuse, 215

esteem needs, in Maslow's hierarchy of needs, 121

euthanasia, 247

exhaustion as response to stress, 161

experience (see educational experience; life experience)

facial expressions, 30

fear (see frightened, angry, aggressive clients)

feedback from communication, 27

fight or flight response to stress, 160–161

foreign languages, 34–35

formal-operations period of development, in cognitive development theory, 83

Freud, Sigmund, in psychoanalytical development theory, 89, 90

frightened, angry, aggressive clients, 147–156

  agoraphobia, 150

  angry/aggressive clients, 150–153

  controlling your own hostility, 153

  destructive behavior, 152–153

  documenting behavior, 153

  frightened clients, 148–149

  inappropriate aggressive behavior, 147

  panic attacks, 150

  phobias, 150

  responding to client's anger, 152

  responding to client's fears, 149–150

General Adaptation Syndrome (GAS), 160

generativity vs. stagnation stage, in psychoanalytical development theory, 97, 103

genetic influences, 7

genital stage , in psychosexual development, 94

genuineness, in helping interviews, 45, 49

gestures & mannerisms, 33, 35

grieving or dying clients, 237–250

  acceptance, 240

  adolescents and grief, 241

  adults and grief, 241

  Advance Directives, 245–246

  anger, 239

  anticipatory grief, 238, 242

  bargaining, 239

  children and grief, 241

  cultural differences in dealing with loss, 237, 240

  denial, 239

  depression, 240

  dysfunctional grief, 238, 243

  elder adults and grief, 241

  Engle's processes of grief, 237, 239

  euthanasia, 247

  factors influencing grief, 237, 241–242

  family members and grief, 237

  gender differences in grief response, 237, 241–242

  Hemlock Society, 246

  hospice, 246

  kinds of losses, 237, 240–241

  Kubler-Ross's stages of grief and dying, 237, 239–240

  life-threatening illnesses, 243–244

  Living Will, 246

  Patient Self-Determination Act, 246

  physician-assisted suicide, 246–247

  Physician's Directive, 238, 246

  right to die laws, 245–247

  terminal illnesses, 243–244

  therapeutic response to grief and dying, 245

guilt, 96, 101

helping interview, 45–68

  acknowledging feelings, 51

  advice & approval, 46, 55

  belittling, contradicting, criticizing, 46, 56

  changing the subject, 46, 57

  clarifying & validating, 51

  clichés & stereotypical responses, 46, 55

  closed questions, 46, 53, 67

  closing the interview, 46

  components of an interview, 46–47

  control factor in successful interview, 47

  defending, 46, 57

  feelings experienced by helper vs. those helped, 45

genuineness, 45, 49

identification of client's problem, 46, 50–52

indirect statements, 46, 54, 67

journaling exercise, 66

levels of need, 46, 52, 66, **53**

moralizing & lecturing, 57–58

open-ended questions, 46, 53–54, 67

orientation of professional and client to each other, 46, 48–49, 62

preparing for the interview, 45

questioning techniques, 52–54

reflecting & paraphrasing, 51–52

requesting explanation of behavior, 46, 55–56

resolution of client's problem, 46, 58–61

responding skills, 46, 64, 65

risk/trust, 45, 49, 63

roadblocks to communication, 46, 54–58, 67

shaming or threatening, 58

sharing observations, 50, **51**

sincerity, 46, 50

sympathy & empathy, 46, 50

Trust Walk exercise, 63

warmth & caring, 45, 49

Hemlock Society, 246

hidden areas of self-perception, Johari window, 12–13

hierarchy of needs, 119–121, **120**

HIV (see AIDS clients)

Holmes, Thomas H., 157, 162

homeostasis, in Maslow's hierarchy of needs, 120

hospice, 246
  AIDS, 232

How to Help a Friend, 52

human relations skills, 3, 4–6

humanism (see behavioral and humanistic development), 115

hypochondria, 179

I Am statements, exercise, 19

id, in psychoanalytical development theory, 89, 90

ideal self, 3, 11–12, 20

identification of client's problem, in helping interviews, 46, 50–52

identification, as defense mechanism, 69, 73

identify vs. role confusion stage, in psychoanalytical development theory, 97, 102, 103

incest, 219

independent lifestyles, elder adults and therapeutic communication, 138

indirect statements, in helping interviews, 46, 54, 67

industry vs. inferiority stage, in psychoanalytical development theory, 97, 102, 103

inferiority, 97, 102, 103

initiative vs. guilt stage , in psychoanalytical development theory, 96, 101

instrumental conditioning, in behavioral theory, 118

integrity vs. despair stage, in psychoanalytical development theory, 98, 103

intentionality, in moral development theory, 108

internal milieu, 8, 159

intimacy vs. isolation stage, in psychoanalytical development theory, 97, 103

intuitive stage of development, in cognitive development theory, 82

involutional depression, 175, 179

isolation, 97, 103

jargon, 134

Jellinek, E.M., 206

Johari Window, 3, 12–13, **13, 14**

journaling exercise, 66

keys to successful communication, 23, 29–30

kinesics, 23, 29

Kohlberg, Lawrence, 107, 109

Kübler-Ross, Elisabeth, 239–240

Landau reflex, 100

latent stage , in psychosexual
    development, 94

leadership qualities, 24, 36
    authoritarian leaders, 24, 36
    Management By Wandering Around
        (MBWA), 24, 36
    Maslow's Hierarchy of Needs, 36
    participative leaders, 24, 36

learning theories
    behavioral and humanistic theories, 115–124
    cognitive development, 79–87
    moral development, 107–114
    psychoanalytic development, 89–106
    social learning theory, 119

levels of need, in helping interviews, 46, 52,
    66, **53**

life experience, 8

life-threatening illnesses, 243–244

limits, adolescents and therapeutic commu-
    nication, 132

listening skills, 24, 36–39, 130

Living Will, 246

management (see leadership qualities)

Management By Wandering Around
    (MBWA), 24, 36

manic depression, 175, 179–180

Maslow, Abraham, 119–121

Maslow's Hierarchy of Needs, 36, 119–121,
    120

melancholia, 179

*Mental Health Nursing, A Holistic
    Approach*, 215

mentors (see models & mentors)

message in communications, 26–27

middle-age crisis, 97, 103

misinterpreting nonverbal communications,
    33–34, 33

mistrust, 95 , 98–100

models & mentors, 9

modes of communications, 23

moral development
    conventional level, 109, 110
    encouraging healthy lifestyles and moral
        development, 107, 110–111
    influences on moral development, 107
    intentionality, 108
    Kohlberg's stages of moral development,
        107, 109–110
    naturalistic behavior, 109
    Piaget's dimensions of moral develop-
        ment, 107, 108
    postconventional (principled) level,
        109, 110
    preconventional level, 109, 110
    premoral level, 110
    principled level, 109, 110
    punishment, 108–109
    reciprocity, 108
    relativism, 108
    restitution, 108–109
    sanctions, 108
    stages of moral development, 107

morality (see values and morals)

moralizing & lecturing, in helping inter-
    views, 57–58

music (see electronic media influences)

narcotics, in drug abuse, 208

naturalistic behavior, in moral development theory, 109

negative characteristics, modifying, 4, 15–16, 21

negative reinforcement, in behavioral theory, 115, 118

nonverbal communications, 23, 29–34, 41

  clustering of nonverbal cues, 30

  congruency between verbal and nonverbal message, 29–30

  facial expressions, 30

  gestures & mannerisms, 33, 35

  kinesics, 29

  misinterpreting nonverbal communications, 33–34

  posture & position in communication, 32–33

  territoriality in communication, 31–32, 40, **31**

  touch as communication, 30–31

Oedipal stage, in psychosexual development, 94

open areas of self-perception, Johari window, 12–13

open-ended questions, in helping interviews, 46, 53–54, 67

operant conditioning, in behavioral theory, 118

oral stage of psychosexual development, 93

orientation of professional and client to each other, in helping interviews, 46, 48–49, 62

overprotectiveness, elder adults and therapeutic communication, 138

panic attacks, 150, 164

paranoid ideation, 179

paraphrasing, and repeating communications, 37, 51–52

Parents Anonymous, 222

participative leaders, 24, 36

Patient Self-Determination Act, 246

Pavlov, Ivan, 115, 116–117

perception of self, 3

personal space, 31–32, 40, **31**

phallic/Oedipal stage , in psychosexual development, 94

phobias, 150

physical dependency on drugs/alcohol, 204

physician-assisted suicide, 246–247

Physician's Directive, 238, 246

Piaget, Jean, 79, 80–81, 107, 108

pleasure principle , in psychoanalytical development theory, 90

positive characteristics, 21

positive reinforcement, in behavioral theory, 115, 118

postconventional (principled) level, in moral development theory, 109, 110

postpartum depression, 181–182

postcrisis phase of violence, in abuse, 216

post-traumatic stress syndrome, 71

posture & position in communication, 32–33

preconceptual stage of development, in cognitive development theory, 82

preconventional level, in moral development theory, 109, 110

premoral level, in moral development theory, 110

preoperational period of development, in cognitive development theory, 82

preventive health care, 134

principled level , in moral development theory, 109, 110

privacy, 133–134

  adolescents and therapeutic communication, 132

  adults and therapeutic communication

Professional Development, 28

projection, as defense mechanism, 69, 72

psychoanalytic development, 89–106

   autonomy vs. shame and doubt stage, 96, 101

   conscience, 91

   ego, 89, 90–91

   ego integrity, 98

   ego psychology, 95

   ego-ideal, 91

   Ericson's stages of psychosocial development, 89, 98–103

   erogenous zones, 89, 92

   Freud's psychosocial forces, 89, 90

   generativity vs. stagnation stage, 97, 103

   id, 89, 90

   identity vs. role confusion stage, 97, 102

   industry vs. inferiority stage, 97, 102

   initiative vs. guilt stage, 96, 101

   integrity vs. despair stage, 98

   intimacy vs. isolation stage, 97, 103

   pleasure principle, 90

   psychosexual development stages, 89, 92–95

   psychosocial crises, 95, 96, 95

   psychosocial forces, 89, 90

   reality principle, 90–91

   reflex responses, 90

   superego, 89, 91

   trust vs. mistrust stage, 95, 98–100

psychosexual development stages, 89, 92–95

   anal stage, 93–94, 93

   genital stage, 94

   latent stage, 94

   oral stage, 93

   phallic/Oedipal stage, 94

psychosocial crises, in psychoanalytical development theory, 95, 96, **95**

psychosocial forces, in psychoanalytical development theory, 89, 90

public self, 3, 11–12, 20

punishment , in behavioral theory, 115, 119

punishment, in moral development theory, 108–109

questioning techniques, in helping interviews, 52–54

racial prejudice & discrimination, 35

Rahe, Richard H., 157, 162

rape, 213, 219–220

rationalization, 69, 74, **74**

reactive depression, 175, 177–178

real self, 3, 11–12, 20

reality principle, in psychoanalytical development theory, 90–91

receiver in communications, 27, **27**

reciprocity, in moral development theory, 108

recovery phase of violence, in abuse, 216

reflecting & paraphrasing, in helping interviews, 51–52

reflex responses , in psychoanalytical development theory, 90

regression, as defense mechanism, 69, 70–71

relativism, in moral development theory, 108

religion (see spirituality & religion)

repression, as defense mechanism, 69, 71

requesting explanation of behavior, in helping interviews, 46, 55–56

resolution of client's problem, in helping interviews, 46, 58–61

respect and dignity

   adolescents and therapeutic communication, 132

   elder adults and therapeutic communication, 138

responding skills, in helping interviews, 46, 64, 65

restitution, in moral development theory, 108–109

return-to-normal stage following stress, 161–162

risk/trust , in helping interviews, 45, 49, 63

roadblocks to effective communications, 24, 46, 54–58, 67

Rogers, Carl, 80, 121

role confusion, 97, 102, 103

role models (see models & mentors)

safety needs, in Maslow's hierarchy of needs, 120

sanctions, in moral development theory, 108

Satir, Virginia, 11, 14

seasonal affective disorder (SAD), 180–181, **181**

self-acceptance, 10

self-actualization , in Maslow's hierarchy of needs, 121

self-analysis, 3, 10–12, 20

self-awareness, 3–22

blind areas of self-perception, Johari window, 12–13

characteristics of successful therapeutic communicators, 16–17

defining self-awareness, 9–11

hidden areas of self-perception, Johari window, 12–13

human relations skills, 3, 4–6

I Am statements, exercise, 19

ideal vs. public vs. real self, 3, 11–12, 20

Johari Window, 3, 12–13, **13, 14**

negative characteristics, modifying, 4, 15–16, 21

open areas of self-perception, Johari window, 12–13

perception of self, 3

positive characteristics, 21

self-acceptance, 10

self-analysis, 3, 10–12

social vs. therapeutic communications, 3, 7–9

technical vs. human relations skills, 6

therapeutic communication, 4–6

uniqueness of each individual, 15

unknown areas of self-perception, Johari window, 12–13

Selye, Hans, 157

sender in communications, 26–27, **27**

sensorimotor period of development, in cognitive development theory, 81–82

sexual abuse, 213, 219

sexuality, adolescents and therapeutic communication, 132

sexually suggestive clients, 197–202

attitudes toward sexuality, 198–199

responding to sexual advances, 200

therapeutic approach to sexual advances, 199–200

shame, 96, 101

shaming or threatening, in helping interviews, 58

sharing observations, in helping interviews, 50, **51**

sincerity , in helping interviews, 46, 50

Skinner, B.F., 115, 116, 118–119

social learning theory, 119

Social Readjustment Scale, 162, 171–172

social vs. therapeutic communications, 3, 7–9

space (see personal space), 31–32, **31**

spirituality & religion, 8–9

spousal abuse, 213, 217

stagnation, 97, 103

stimulants, in drug abuse, 208

stressed and anxious clients, 134, 157–174

adolescents and stress, 166–167

adults and stress, 167–168

alarm as response to stress, 160

anxiety levels, 157, 162–164

Bernard's theory of stress, 159

burnout, 167–168

Cannon's theory of stress, 159–160

children and stress, 164–166

defining stress, 158–159

elder adults and stress, 168

exhaustion as response to stress, 161

fight or flight response to stress, 160–161

General Adaptation Syndrome (GAS), 160

good vs. bad stress, 158–159

internal milieu and stress, 159

life cycle experience of stress, 164–168

panic attacks, 164

reducing stress, 169–170

return-to-normal stage following stress, 161–162

Selye's classification of stress, 160

signs and symptoms of stress, 158, 159, 160–162

Social Readjustment Scale, 162, 171–172

theories of stress, 159–162

web sites for more information, 173

sublimation, as defense mechanism, 69, 72

substance-abusing clients, 203–212

alcoholism, 203, 205–207

cycle of substance abuse, 204, **205**

drug-abuse, 207–210

emotional dependency on drugs/ alcohol, 204

Jellinek's four phases of alcoholism, 203, 206

physical dependency on drugs/ alcohol, 204

risk factors for substance abuse, 204

therapeutic response to alcoholism, 207

suicidal clients, 187–196

evaluating probability, 187

intervention resources, 193

physician-assisted suicide, 246–247

risk factors for suicide, 187, 188–190

statistics on suicide, 188–189

steps and stages of contemplating suicide, 187, 190–191

therapeutic response to suicidal clients, 191–192

verbal vs. nonverbal messages warning suicide, 187, 189, 194

warning signs of suicide, 189–190

web sites for more information, 195

superego, in psychoanalytical development theory, 89, 91

survival/physiological needs, in Maslow's hierarchy of needs, 120

sympathy & empathy, in helping interviews, 46, 50

Taber's Cyclopedic Dictionary, 29

team attitude to health care, 134

team communication, 36

technical vs. human relations skills, 6

technology and communications, 24, 35–36

television (see electronic media influences)

terminal illnesses, 243–244

territoriality in communication, 31–32, 40, **31**

therapeutic process, 9–14

touch as communication, 30–31

transitioning from pediatric to adult care, 132–133

triggering phase of violence, in abuse, 215

trust vs. mistrust stage , in psychoanalytical development theory, 95, 98–100

Trust Walk exercise, 63

undoing, as defense mechanism, 69, 73

uniqueness of each individual, 15

unknown areas of self-perception, Johari
    window, 12–13

values & morals, 9, 91

verbal communications, 28

Victims of Child Abuse Laws (VOCAL), 222

warmth & caring, in helping interviews,
    45, 49

Welter, Paul, 52

Wilkes, Mary, 28

withdrawal symptoms , in drug abuse, 208